ENDOMETRIOSIS
Current Concepts and
Future Directions

METHIL KANNAN KUTTY

MUHAMED T OSMAN

ISBN-13: 978-1500252526
ISBN-10: 1500252522

DEDICATION

This book is dedicated to all patients who have endometriosis.

Kannan and Osman

CONTENTS

PREFACE

The spectacle of amazing advances in the complex spectrum of the etiology, pathogenesis and treatment of gynecological disorders in general and endometriosis in particular provides an exciting venture for all those interested in current trends in gynecology and this is the raison d'etre for this book. Spectacular achievements in the state of the art technology and progressive discoveries such as microRNA etc has impacted all facets of medical disciplines in unraveling molecular mechanisms of diseases including endometriosis. Cognizant of this scenario adorned by the cutting edge of modern technology and its paramount importance in perceptive of the fundamentals of pathogenesis of endometriosis, a common disorder we have dealt with some of the breakthroughs for better comprehension of certain facets that have hitherto remained unclear. Endometriosis is a common gynecological disorder which is in fact a global menacing problem. Endometriosis affects more than 10 per cent of women in the reproductive years, with a peak incidence between the ages of 25 and 35. Although fairly common, it can be puzzling as the symptoms vary greatly in their type and severity. It is one of the commonest causes of pelvic pain and infertility in women worldwide. Commonly, several years may elapse before the diagnosis is made. Some women with sinister advanced disease have minimal pain but experience the sudden grief of discovering that they are infertile. It is also a cause of considerable morbidity and needless to reiterate its major impact on public health. We wish all the readers a salubrious journey through this book and if this book succeeds in providing the readers, be they doctors, postgraduate students, physicians or gynecologists, advantageous journey, we will feel a profound sense of satisfaction and achievement of our objectives of writing this. This book acknowledges appreciatively, sincerely and unreservedly all those responsible in one way or another, for stimulating us with their wisdom, experience and expertise.

Methil Kannan kutty; M.B.B.S., M.D., F.R.C.Path and F.R.C.P.A.

Muhamed T. Osman; M.B.Ch.B., M.Sc., Ph.D.

1 INTRODUCTION

Endometriosis, a common gynecologic disorder, is defined by the occurrence of a tissue resembling uterine endometrium, which is sited in aberrant places other than its anatomical locations. These aberrant endometrial heterotopic islands are composed of glands and stroma and are functionally proficient of responding to exogenous, endogenous, or local hormonal stimuli [1].

The name of the disease comes from the word endometrium, the tissue that lines the uterus. In a woman with endometriosis, this endometrial tissue is found outside the uterus: on the ovaries, on the fallopian tubes, in the abdominal cavity, and at other abnormal sites. This tissue found outside the uterus can respond to the menstrual cycle in the same way the lining of the uterus responds. At the end of the luteal phase of the menstrual cycle, when hormones decline and the uterine lining is shed, endometrial tissue growing outside the uterus will also break apart and bleed. This blood has no place to go, so the surrounding tissue may become inflamed and swollen. Scar tissue can form around the endometriosis sites and develop into areas called implants, nodules, lesions, or growths [2-3].

Endometriosis was described at the turn of the century, as severe lesions such as ovarian "chocolate cysts" [4], and as adenomyosis externa [5-8]. Smaller lesions were already in 1899 described by Russell [9] who wrote, *"On the microscopic study of the ovary, we were astonished to find areas which were an exact prototype of the uterine glands and interglandular connective tissue."*. For the next decades, endometriosis was described as a disorder causing pain and requiring surgery. During that period other localizations [10] were described and endometriosis was reported as an 'accidental' finding during surgery for other gynecological disorders [11-13]. Only after the introduction of endoscopy in the late 1960's black-puckered endometriosis lesions were recognized to be a frequent observation in women with pain and/or infertility. When in the 1980's non-pigmented endometriotic lesions were described [14-16], the observed prevalence of the disease further increased [17-20]. In the nineties, the awareness of deep infiltrating endometriosis increased progressively together with the recognition that this type of endometriosis was not always diagnosed during laparoscopy or surgery, especially not during the previous decades.

The ectopic endometrium has been found in the umbilicus, skin, vagina, vulva, cervix, and perineum, in the inguinal canal, upper abdominal peritoneum and organs (liver, spleen), gastrointestinal tract, urinary system, breasts, diaphragm, pleural cavity, brain, eye, lymph nodes, lung and pericardium [21-22].

Unique cases have also been documented in males [23-24]. Cases of diaphragmatic endometriosis are on record and have been reported in small series [8-10]; more than 100 cases of thoracic endometriosis have been documented in the literatures. [21].

Endometriosis affects 8%-10% of women of reproductive age; in 30% of the women, the condition is linked with primary or secondary infertility. In several instances, endometriosis persists as a minimal or mild disease, or it can resolve on its own. Other cases of endometriosis exhibit severe symptoms that terminate with onset of menopause. However, endometriosis can, reactivate in several postmenopausal women when iatrogenic or endogenous hormones are present.

According to the World Endometriosis Research Foundation, it is estimated that 176 million women globally, and 8.5 million in North America are affected with endometriosis, although the exact prevalence is not known [25]. Most cases of endometriosis are diagnosed in women ages 25-35 years of age, but these women experience an average diagnostic delay of seven years from first presenting with symptoms, so many women have symptoms during their teenage years.

According to the World Endometriosis Research Foundation, the annual healthcare costs of endometriosis are estimated to be $70-95 billion, or potentially $110 billion in the United States alone [26-27].

A staging system has been developed by the America Society of Reproductive Medicine based on the location, depth, size, and amount of endometrial growth found during laparoscopy. The stage sometimes does not correlate with the amount of pain a woman has, the symptoms present, or whether fertility is affected [2].

Stage I = minimal severity

Stage II = mild severity

Stage Ill = moderate severity

Stage IV = severe

Its pathogenesis is controversial, and its capricious morphology seems to signify a continuum of individual presentations and progressions. Many theories exist as to what causes endometriosis, and likely it is a combination of all these factors that not only determines the cause but also the severity of the disease. It is important to consider them all in developing a treatment strategy for patients.

Endometriosis has no characteristic signs or symptoms; hence the difficulty in its diagnosis [1]. The cause of endometriosis is unknown. According to Endometriosis.org, the global forum on the disease, most scientists working in the field do believe that endometriosis is exacerbated by estrogen, and there are many theories that have been accepted, and sometimes should be combined to explain the complexity of the disease [28].

The most common symptom of endometriosis is pelvic pain. The pain often correlates to the menstrual cycle, however a woman with endometriosis may also experience pain at other times during her monthly cycle. For many women, but not everyone, the pain of endometriosis can unfortunately be so severe and debilitating that it impacts on her life so that she may not be able to carry out day to day activities [28-29].

Pregnancy occurs when an egg is released from an ovary, travels through the fallopian tube, becomes fertilized by a sperm cell, and attaches itself to the uterine wall to begin development. Endometriosis can obstruct the fallopian tube and keep the egg and sperm from uniting. However, in most cases it is not yet understood why it is harder for women with endometriosis to become pregnant. It is somewhat a myth that women with endometriosis are infertile, but it is reality that 30-40% of them are more likely to have trouble conceiving.

For many women, it can take years to get a diagnosis. That this is because no one symptom or set of symptoms can definitely confirm a diagnosis of endometriosis, however, the symptoms of endometriosis are common and could be caused by a number of other conditions such as irritable bowel syndrome and pelvic inflammatory disease. In addition those different women have different symptoms and some women have no symptoms at all.

There is no simple test for endometriosis. The only way to make a definite diagnosis is by laparoscopy.

Endometriosis is treated by pain-relieving drugs, hormone treatments and surgery which can be used to remove areas of endometriosis. Standard medical therapies for patients with endometriosis include analgesics (nonsteroidal anti-inflammatory drugs [NSAIDs] or acetaminophen), oral contraceptive pills (OCPs), androgenic agents, [30] progestogens, gonadotropin- releasing hormone analogues. However, the surgical treatment includes laparoscopic surgery with ablation of endometrial deposits, hysterectomy and bilateral salpingoooophorectomy [31-32].

The natural history of endometriosis suggests that the disease may stabilize or resolve on its own. Endometriosis may recur after surgery whether or not the patients are treated with estrogen replacement [32-34].

References

1. Acién P, Velasco I. Endometriosis: a disease that remains enigmatic. ISRN Obstet Gynecol. 2013:17:242.

2. Marianne Marchese. Endometriosis. Townsend Letter 2009; April: 59-62

3. Frackiewicz E.J. Endometriosis: an overview of the disease and its treatment. I AM Pharm Assoc. 2000; 40(5):645-657.

4. Sampson JA. Peritoneal endometriosis due to the menstrual dissemination of endometrial tissue into the peritoneal cavity. Am.J.Obstet.Gynecol. 1927;14:422-69.

5. Cullen TS. Adeno-myoma of the round ligament. Johns Hopkins

Hosp.Bull. 1896; 7:112-14.

6. Lockyer, C. Adenomyoma in the recto-uterine and recto-vaginal septa. Proc Royal Soc Med 1913; 6:112-120.

7. Cullen, T. S. The distribution of adenomyomata containing uterine mucosa. Am.J.Obstet.Gynecol. 1919; 80:130-138.

8. Meighs V. An interest in endometriosis and its consequences. Am.J.Obstet.Gynecol. 1920; 79:625.

9. Russell WW. Aberrant portions of the Mullerian duct found in an ovary. Johns Hopkins Hosp.Bull. 1899;94-96:8-10.

10. Latcher, J. W. Endometriosis of the umbilicus. Am.J.Obstet.Gynecol. 1953; 66, 161.

11. Gruenwald P. Origin of endometriosis from the mesenchyme of the celomic walls. Am.J.Obstet.Gynecol. 1942;44:470-74.

12. Scott, R. B. and Telinde, R. W. External endometriosis - the scourge of the private patient. Ann.Surg. 1950;131, 697.

13. Burgmeister RE, Fechner RE, Franklin RR. Endosalpingiosis of the peritoneum. Obstet.Gynecol. 1969; 34:310-17.

14. Jansen RPS, Russel P. Nonpigmented endometriosis: Clinical, laparoscopic, and pathologic definition. Am.J.Obstet.Gynecol. 1986;155:1154-59.

15. Stripling MC, Martin DC, Poston WM. Does endometriosis have a typical appearance? J Reprod Med Obstet.Gynecol. 1988;33:879-84.

16. Martin DC, Hubert GD, Van der Zwaag R, El Zeky FA. Laparoscopic appearances of peritoneal endometriosis. Fertil.Steril. 1989;51:63-67.

17. Mahmood TA, Templeton A. Prevalence and genesis of endometriosis. Hum.Reprod. 1991;6:544- 49.

18. Houston DE, Noller KL, Melton LJ, Selwyn BJ, Hardy RJ. Incidence of pelvic endometriosis in Rochester, Minnesota, 1970- 1979. Am.J.Epidemiol. 1987;125:959-69. Epidemiology of endometriosis *1-5-2003 10*

19. Hull MGR, Glazener CMA, Kelly NJ, et al. Population study of causes, treatment, and outcome of infertility. BMJ. 1985;291:1693-97.

20. Bitzer J, Korber HR. Laparoscopy findings in infertile women. Geburtshilfe.Frauenheilkd. 1983;43:294-98.

21. Jubanyik KJ, Comite F. Extrapelvic endometriosis. Obstet Gynecol Clin North Am 1997; 24: 411-40.

22. Sensenig DM, Serlin O, Hawthorne HR. Pericardial endometriosis. An experimental study in dogs. JAMA 1966; 198: 645-7.

23. Wolthuis AM, Aelvoet C, Bosteels J, Vanrijkel JP. Diaphragmatic endometriosis: diagnosis and surgical management – a case report. Acta Chir Belg 2003; 103: 519-20.

24. Nahir Eldar-Geva T, Alberton J, Beller U. Symptomatic diaphragmatic endometriosis ten years after total abdominal hysterectomy. Obstet Gynecol 2004; 104: 1149-51.

25. Takeuchi H, Kitade M, Sakurai A, et al. Fitz-Hugh and Curtis syndrome-like diaphragmatic endometriosis. Fertil Steril 2005; 83: 1039-40.

26. Cucinella G, Granese R, Calagna G, et al. Laparoscopic treatment of diaphragmatic endometriosis causing chronic shoulder and arm pain. Acta Obstet Gynecol Scand 2009; 88: 1418-9.

27. Gilalbert-Estelles J, Zorio E, Castello JM, et al. Laparoscopic approach to right diaphragmatic endometriosis with argon laser: case report. J Minim Invasive Gynecol 2010; 17: 124-7.

28. World Endometriosis Research Foundation. "Facts about endometriosis" http://endometriosisfoundation.org/Facts-about-endometriosis.pdf

29. Impact of Endometriosis.

http://www.womeningovernment.org/files/LoneHummel.pdf

30. S. Simoens, L. Hummelshoj, and T. D'Hooghe. Human Reproduction Update, Vol.13, No.4 pp. 395–404, 2007, Endometriosis: cost estimates and methodological perspective.
http://humupd.oxfordjournals.org/content/13/4/395.full.pdf

31. Endometriosis.org.The Global Forum on Endometriosis. "Causes"

http://endometriosis.org/endometriosis/causes/. Accessed on 12th March 2014.

32. Selak V, Farquhar C, Prentice A, Singla A. Danazol for pelvic pain associated with endometriosis. Cochrane Database Syst Rev 2001; (4):CD000068.

33. Namnoum AB, Hickman TN, Goodman SB, Gehlbach DL, Rock JA. Incidence of symptom recurrence after hysterectomy for endometriosis. Fertil Steril 1995;64:898-902.

34. Anne L. Mounsey, Alex Wilgus, David C. Slawson. Diagnosis and Management of Endometriosis. American Family Physician 2006; 74(4): 595-601.

2 EPIDEMIOLOGY OF ENDOMETRIOSIS

The exact prevalence of endometriosis is not known since a laparoscopy is required to make the diagnosis and since the recognition varies with the training and the interest of the laparoscopist. Moreover the pathophysiology is poorly understood, which makes it difficult to formulate and test simple hypotheses [1].

The definitions of endometriosis have changed over time, contributing to biases in the literature. In the mid eighties, the non pigmented or subtle endometriosis was introduced, and from the nineties onwards the recognition of deep endometriosis has progressively increased.

The revised American Fertility Society (rAFS) classification is widely used. Yet we have to recognize that this classification has never been validated as a classification for pain or infertility. Taken together, the absence of an easy non-invasive diagnosis, the changing definitions, and the absence of a clear understanding of the pathophysiology and the absence of a validated classification system, is the cause that still today the endometriosis literature is full of confusion [1].

In the 1980's, the prevalence of the disease increased from 5% to 20% to over 60% to 80% in women with infertility and/or pelvic pain [1-3].

The prevalence clearly increases with the awareness and the training of the surgeon. In all series the underlying biases of no confirmation or at best limited confirmation by pathology should be recognized.

The prevalence of subtle lesions decreases with age for unknown reasons [3-4]. No studies are available demonstrating a clear association with any of the variables considered important such as early menarche, short cycles, abundant or painful periods, subfertility, canalization defects of the cervix, race, dioxin, total body radiation, or any other factor.

Assuming that typical endometriosis contributes predominantly, to the reported prevalences of endometriosis, the prevalences in a clinic populations vary from about a 4% occurrence of largely asymptomatic endometriosis found in women undergoing tubal ligation to 50% of teenagers with intractable dysmenorrhea. Prevalences in women with pain or infertility range between 40 to 70% [3, 5].

General population incidence during the 1970s in the USA has been suggested to be 1.6 per 1000 white females aged 15-49, while a more current study based upon hospital discharges finds endometriosis as a first listed diagnosis in 1.3 per 1000 discharges in women aged 15-44. [6]

In a large study comprising all women in an area in Norway the lifetime risk for endometriosis was 2.2% [7]. In this study, early menarche, frequent menstruations, pelvic pain, infertility and nulliparity are associated with endometriosis. In a controlled study of women with infertility and a normal partner, compared with women with an azoospermic partner, stage I endometriosis is not more common in infertile women than in an unselected women. However, stage II disease endometriosis was more frequent, (3.3% vs. 5.7%t) in infertile women. [8]

There is a non validated clinical impression that endometriosis could vary with the race, blacks having lower rates of endometriosis and Orientals have higher rates than whites.

Endometriosis is clearly associated with dysmenorrhea, but it is unknown whether this is a cause or a consequence.

Dioxin pollution has been suggested to be causally related to endometriosis. This hypothesis, formulated in 1994 [9] based upon indirect observations, became popular following the observation that the incidence and the severity of endometriosis increased in primates treated previously with dioxins [10-11]. In the human final proof is still lacking. [12].

Breast-fed infants, possibly exposed to dioxins in milk, moreover have unexpectedly a lower incidence of endometriosis in adult life. [13]

Total body radiation is associated with increased prevalence of endometriosis in primates [14].

Endometriosis clearly is a hereditary disease. [15-16] The prevalence of first degree relatives is some 7 times higher than in control groups. In monozygotic twins the prevalence is even up to 15 times higher.

The lower natural killer cell activity in plasma and in peritoneal fluid [17-20], has fueled speculation about the role of the immune system and endometriosis [21]. Until today, however, no clear association is found between endometriosis prevalence and chronic immunosuppression, e.g. in transplant patients, nor with smoking affecting NK activity, nor with caffeine or alcohol, nor with any lifestyle variable.

Stress could be causally related to endometriosis. This concept is derived from the association of endometriosis and LUF syndrome, of an association between a higher trait anxiety and LUF syndrome [22-23], and of the hypothesis that the lower steroid hormone concentrations in peritoneal fluid might favour the implantation/development of endometriosis [24]. This hypothesis can, however, not be tested since there is no adequate animal model.

Another argument to link endometriosis and stress is the widely held belief that endometriosis is a career women's disease. This, however, can equally well be explained by the delay of childbearing in this group of women, with the inevitable increase of infertility with age, and a higher prevalence of endometriosis at laparoscopy.

Nulliparity could be a consequence of the disease but in a large study in Italy the prevalence decreased with increasing parity. [25]

Oral contraception use has been reported to be associated with a decreased prevalence [26].

Endometriosis was suggested to be associated with an increased risk in ovarian cancer (OR = 1.73, 95% CI: 1.10, 2.71) [27], and of non Hodgkin lymphoma [28]

Cystic ovarian endometriosis increases with age [25]. Most reports confirmed that cystic ovarian endometriosis is clonal in origin. [29-30]

Deep endometriosis increases with age [3]. Rectovaginal endometriosis was known since the beginning of the century, but the high prevalence of deep endometriosis remained unsuspected until fairly recently. In the population these conditions, were considered relatively rare but actually estimates of prevalence of 3 to 10% seem appropriate. This estimation of some 10% to 20% deep endometriosis is derived from observations in Leuven from 1988 to 1991 [3], a period during which endoscopic surgery was not yet well developed, and in which deep endometriosis was not yet a well known entity. Referrals were thus only those for infertility and pain not for deep endometriosis. Assuming that laparoscopies for infertility are performed in some 10% to 15% of the population and taking into account that Leuven is a tertiary referral center, the prevalence of deep endometriosis can be estimated to be between 1% (the prevalence is 10% in younger age group with infertility which can be estimated at 15% of the population; in a tertiary center the prevalence is probably slightly overestimated) and 3% (prevalence of 20% of the older age group with infertility). Taking into account the observation that by menstrual clinical examination deep endometriosis is more frequent, prevalences between 3% and 10% seem a fair estimate [1].

Indeed the exact prevalence of endometriosis in any one country is difficult to predict with any degree of accuracy due to the invasive and subjective diagnostic procedures required to diagnose endometriosis. Although non-invasive methods for detecting endometriosis are currently under development, such as the CA125 antigen test [31], ultrasound scanning [32] and endometrial nerve density [33], definitive diagnosis of endometriosis can only be achieved visually via laparoscopy. However, diagnosis is a subjective matter depending on the skill of the surgeon and the quality of equipment used. Therefore, in poorer countries prevalence rates of endometriosis may be under represented due to lack of specialized doctors and poor quality surgical equipment. The 10% figure is often quoted as a universal constant for endometriosis prevalence. This may be erroneous however, given the heterogeneity of the world's populations the prevalence of endometriosis is likely to vary widely. Like many other diseases, prevalence of endometriosis will vary throughout the world but without a simple, objective diagnostic method the true prevalence of endometriosis within certain populations cannot be accurately measured. Endometriosis is a multifactoral disease, meaning it is highly unlikely a singular causative factor will ever be found. Like certain cancer types lifetime endometriosis risk is influenced by a number of factors. However, from the few epidemiological studies that have assessed endometriosis, certain factors can be used as indicators for the likelihood of endometriosis arising in populations where those factors are known. For example, the epidemiological data on endometriosis suggests that women with high parity, low meat consumption, high fruit and vegetable consumption, low alcohol consumption and live in a rural environment are less likely to develop endometriosis than those who have low parity, high meat consumption etc [34-35]. Additionally, women with endometriosis have been shown to have an increased risk of developing ovarian cancer [36]. The reason for this is thought to be due to endometriosis of the ovary representing a pre-malignant state in some cases [37-38]. Whilst the prevalence of endometriosis in most of the world's countries may not be known, data on known mentioned risk factors is well documented for most countries.

There were some attempts had been made to identify women at increased risk by means of a variety of demographic correlates [39-40]. Certain personality traits (achieving, egocentric, overanxious, perfectionist, intelligent) and body build (underweight) have been reported with increased frequency in affected women.

The validity of such observations has not been established. Studies did not find a particular group of patients to be more susceptible to endometriosis.

These findings support the suggestion that there is no particular personality trait or ethnic predilection in this disease [39].

The true incidence of endometriosis is difficult to establish since endoscopy or laparotomy is required for definitive diagnosis and the disease undoubtedly exists in many patients who do not have symptoms that lead to a surgical procedure. There seems to be a racial, social and geographic distribution of endometriosis. For example, a study [41] has reported an exceptionally low incidence of 1.12% in a unique ultra-orthodox Jewish population over the past 20 years by reviewing 1434 hysterectomy specimens. These findings may suggest the possible effects of heredity, religious and social behaviour on the etiology of endometriosis. It is generally believed that the disease is relatively less common in India, Pakistan, Iran, countries of the Middle East, and Black Africa [42]. However, these observations are merely variations in clinical impression. No solid data exist to support this contention. On the contrary, a few reports which are available from these countries seem to refute it. [39].

The clinical impression of low incidence of endometriosis in Asian and black women may have been due to limited medical and diagnostic facilities available to these women. With the improvement of these facilities, and wider use of surgical interventions in these patients, more and more endometriosis cases will undoubtedly be detected. For example, incidence of endometriosis was found to be high in Iran [43], black women in America [44], in Japanese women in Hawaii and Japan [45], Chinese women in Taiwan [39, 46], and in Caucasian women in Italy [47] . In other Asian study the incidence of association of endometriosis with infertility is relatively higher and may be a reflection of selection bias as already noted in other countries [39].

Prevalence corresponds to, and increases with, awareness and training of the surgeon, but endometriosis is estimated to affect nearly 176 million women globally; 775,000 in Canada and 8.5 million in North America overall [48-49]. Mistakenly once believed to be a disease of older women, nearly 70% of teens with pelvic pain are later diagnosed with endometriosis [50]. Early intervention and increased awareness is requisite to reduce morbidity, infertility, and progressive symptomatology in patients of all ages.

Parity and infertility have long been associated with endometriosis, with infertility among the chief clinical findings. As well, associated pain, anatomic distortion, development of adhesions, altered inflammatory response characterized by neovascularization and fibrosis formation, abnormal T- and B-cell functionality, abnormal complement deposition, and altered interleukin-6 are among clinical consequences [51]. Endometriosis is also clearly associated with dysmenorrhea, but it is unknown whether this is a cause or a consequence [48, 52].

There is no known disease prevention. Related to a number of hereditary, environmental, epigenetic, and menstrual characteristics and alterations, some sharing certain common processes with cancer, [53] endometriosis remains the third leading cause of gynecologic hospitalization in United States [54] and is considered a leading cause of female primary and secondary infertility, prevalent in 0.5% to 5.0% in fertile and 25% to 40% of infertile women. [30] The disease is also a leading cause of hysterectomy in the United States, with significant associated morbidity. [55]

Though no particular demographic, personality trait, or ethnic predilection has been defined, certain characteristics have been associated with diagnosis, including decreased risk with late age at menarche [56] and shorter menstrual cycles with longer duration of flow. [57]

Likewise, family history cannot be undervalued, with consistent findings illustrating a near 10-fold increased risk in those women with first-degree relatives who have endometriosis. [58] Further genetic analyses will clarify the role of family in disease risk [48].

Dioxin pollution has been suggested to be causally related to endometriosis based on the observation of increased incidence and severity of disease in primates treated previously with dioxins. [59] Related data suggest plausibility that dioxin exposure of specific timing and dosage may precipitate endometriosis through interaction with estrogen receptors or suppression of progesterone receptors [60]. Conversely, at least one more recent study concluded that dioxin may not contribute to the etiology of endometriosis at all. [61]

No clear association has been defined between endometriosis prevalence and chronic immunosuppression, for example, in transplant patients, nor with smoking affecting NK activity, nor with caffeine or alcohol, nor with any lifestyle variable [52]. Studies have found that higher body mass index decreases risk of both deep as well as ovarian and pelvic endometriosis, as does parity, [62] though pregnancy is not a cure [48].

Frequency of endometriosis in women of higher social class has been reported, but this is likely the result of bias. The same diagnostic bias may explain the higher frequency in white women versus women of color, and in fact, data on prevalence in different races often do not consider the reason for admission for surgical procedure, which may be selectively associated with a higher or lower likelihood of an endometriosis diagnosis. Few studies have evaluated comparable population and socioeconomic conditions; those that did revealed no substantial differences among women of different races [60]. Less understood are the factors, if any, of nutrition and exercise, lifestyle, personality traits, and other variables, with little evidence regarding these as more than simply modulating roles [48].

Data on specific phenotypic traits of women with the disease are also sparse. However, in a recent provocative study by Vercellini and colleagues [63] determined that women with the most severe form of endometriosis appeared more attractive to external observers than those with peritoneal and/or ovarian endometriosis, as well as those without endometriosis. Women with severe rectovaginal disease were judged to have a leaner silhouette, larger breasts, and a history of earlier coitarche. Whilst phenotyping may have future use in conjunction with genetic and environmental data to elucidate the pathogenesis of endometriosis, the authors did caution that further studies are warranted to "exclude a spurious relationship between attractiveness and rectovaginal endometriosis and to rule out the potentially confounding effect of deep dyspareunia on some aspects of sexual behavior." [48].

References

1. Philippe R. Koninckz, Anastasia Ussia. Epidemiology of endometriosis. Book chapter written April 2003;5: 1-16.

2. Bitzer J, Korber HR. Laparoscopy findings in infertile women. Geburtshilfe.Frauenheilkd. 1983;43:294-98.

3. Koninckx PR, Meuleman C, Demeyere S, Lesaffre E, Cornillie FJ. Suggestive evidence that pelvic endometriosis is a progressive disease, whereas deeply infiltrating endometriosis is associated with pelvic pain. Fertil.Steril. 1991;55:759-65.

4. Redwine DB. Age-related evolution in color appearance of endometriosis. Fertil.Steril. 1987;48:1062-63.

5. Walter AJ, Hentz JG, Magtibay PM, Cornella JL, Magrina JF. Endometriosis: correlation between histologic and visual findings at laparoscopy. Am.J.Obstet.Gynecol. 2001;184:1407-11.

6. Cramer DW, Missmer SA. The epidemiology of endometriosis. Ann.N.Y.Acad.Sci. 2002;955:11- 22.

7. Moen, M. H. and Schei, B. Epidemiology of endometriosis in a Norwegian county. Acta Obstet.Gynecol.Scand. 76(6), 559-562. 1997.

8. Matorras R, Rodriguez F, Pijoan JI, Etxanojauregui A, Neyro JL, Elorriaga MA et al. Women who are not exposed to spermatozoa and infertile women have similar rates of stage I endometriosis. Fertil.Steril. 2001;76:923-28.

9. Koninckx PR, Braet P, Kennedy SH, Barlow DH. Dioxin pollution and endometriosis in Belgium [see comments]. Hum.Reprod. 1994;9:1001- 02.

10. Rier SE, Martin DC, Bowman RE, Dmowski WP, Becker JL. Endometriosis in Rhesus Monkeys (Macaca-mulatta) Following Chronic Exposure to 2,3,7,8-Tetrachlorodibenzo-p-dioxin. Fund.Appl.Toxicol. 1993;21:433-41.

11. Rier SE, Turner WE, Martin DC, Morris R, Lucier GW, Clark GC. Serum levels of TCDD and dioxin-like chemicals in Rhesus monkeys chronically exposed to dioxin: correlation of increased serum PCB levels with endometriosis. Toxicol.Sci. 2001;59:147-59.

12. Koninckx PR. The physiopathology of endometriosis: pollution and dioxin. Gynecol.Obstet.Invest 1999;47 Suppl 1:47-49.

13. Tsutsumi O, Momoeda M, Takai Y, Ono M, Taketani Y. Breast-fed infants, possibly exposed to dioxins in milk, have unexpectedly lower incidence of endometriosis in adult life. Int.J.Gynaecol.Obstet. 2000;68:151-53.

14. Fanton JW, Golden JG. Radiation-induced endometriosis in Macaca mulatta. Radiat.Res. 1991;126:141-46

15. Kennedy SH, Mardon H, Barlow DH. Familial endometriosis. J.Assist.Reprod.Genet. 1995;12:32- 34.

16. Hadfield, R. M., Mardon, H. J., Barlow, D. H., and Kennedy, S. H. Endometriosis in monozygotic twins. Fertil.Steril. 68(5), 941-942. 1997.

17. Cornillie FJ, Oosterlynck D, Lauweryns JM, Koninckx PR. Deeply infiltrating pelvic endometriosis: histology and clinical significance. Fertil.Steril. 1990;53:978-83.

18. Oosterlynck D. Immunosuppressive activity of peritoneal fluid in women with endometriosis. Obstet.Gynecol. 1993;82:206-12.

19. Oosterlynck DJ, Meuleman C, Waer M, Koninckx PR. Transforming Growth Factor-beta Activity Is Increased in Peritoneal Fluid from Women with Endometriosis. Obstet.Gynecol. 1994;83:287- 92.

20. Oosterlynck DJ, Meuleman C, Waer M, Koninckx PR, Vandeputte M. Immunosuppressive activity of peritoneal fluid in women with endometriosis. Obstet.Gynecol. 1993;82:206-12.

21. Braun D, Ding J, Shen J, Rana N, Fernandez B, Dmowski W. Relationship between apoptosis and the number of macrophages in eutopic endometrium from women with and without endometriosis. Fertil.Steril. 2002;78:830.

22. Koninckx PR. Pelvic endometriosis: A consequence of stress? Contrib.Gynecol.Obstet. 1987;16:56-59.

23. Demyttenaere K, Nijs P, Evers-Kiebooms G, Koninckx PR. Coping and the ineffectiveness of coping influence the outcome of in vitro fertilization through stress responses. Psychoneuroendocrinology. 1992;17:655-65.

24. Koninckx PR, Kennedy SH, Barlow DH. Pathogenesis of endometriosis: The role of peritoneal fluid. Gynecol.Obstet.Invest. 1999;47 Suppl. 1:23-33.

25. Parazzini F, Luchini L, Vezzoli F, Mezzanotte C, Vercellini P, Romanini C et al. Prevalence and anatomical distribution of endometriosis in women with selected gynaecological conditions: Results from a multicentric Italian study. Hum.Reprod. 1994;9:1158-62.

26. Mahmood TA, Templeton A. Prevalence and genesis of endometriosis. Hum.Reprod. 1991;6:544- 49.

27. Ness RB, Cramer DW, Goodman MT, Kjaer SK, Mallin K, Mosgaard BJ et al. Infertility, fertility drugs, and ovarian cancer: a pooled analysis of case-control studies. Am.J.Epidemiol. 2002;155:217-24.

28. Olson JE, Cerhan JR, Janney CA, Anderson KE, Vachon CM, Sellers TA. Postmenopausal cancer risk after self-reported endometriosis diagnosis in the Iowa Women's Health Study. Cancer 2002;94:1612-18.

29. Yano T, Jimbo H, Yoshikawa H, Tsutsumi O, Taketani Y. Molecular analysis of clonality in ovarian endometrial cysts. Gynecol.Obstet.Invest. 1999;47 Suppl. 1:41-45.

30. Tamura M, Fukaya T, Murakami I, Uehara S, Yajima A. Analysis of clonality in human endometriotic cysts based on evaluation of X

chromosome inactivation in archival formalin-fixed, paraffin-embedded tissue. Laboratory Investigation 1998;78:213-18.

31. Agic, A., et al., Combination of CCR1 mRNA, MCP1, and CA125 measurements in peripheral blood as a diagnostic test for endometriosis. Reprod Sci, 2008;15(9): 906-11.

32. Volpi, E., et al., Role of transvaginal sonography in the detection of endometriomata. J Clin Ultrasound, 1995;23(3): 163-7.

33. Al-Jefout, M., et al., Diagnosis of endometriosis by detection of nerve fibres in an endometrial biopsy: a double blind study. Hum Reprod, 2009.

34. Fjerbaek, A. and U.B. Knudsen, Endometriosis, dysmenorrhea and diet--what is the evidence? Eur J Obstet Gynecol Reprod Biol, 2007; 132(2):140-7.

35. Parazzini, F., et al., Selected food intake and risk of endometriosis. Hum Reprod, 2004; 19(8): 1755-9.

36. Brinton, L.A., et al., Cancer risk after a hospital discharge diagnosis of endometriosis. Am J Obstet Gynecol, 1997;176(3): 572-9.

37. Vlahos, N.F., T. Kalampokas, and S. Fotiou, Endometriosis and ovarian cancer: A review. Gynecol Endocrinol, 2009: 1-7.

38. Ness, R.B., Endometriosis and ovarian cancer: thoughts on shared pathophysiology. Am J Obstet Gynecol, 2003; 189(1):280-94.

39. Naseer-ud-Din, Ataullah Khan and Nudrat Illahi. Prevalence and presentation of endometriosis in patients admitted in Nishtar Hospital, Multan. JAMC 2000; 12 (3): 22-25

40. Weed JC, Arquembourg PC: Endometriosis: Can it produce an autoimmune response resulting in infertility? Clin Obstet Gynaecol 1980; 23: 885.

41. Simpson JL, Ellas S, Mallnak LR et al: Heritable aspects of endometriosis.Genetic studies. Am J Obstet Gynaecol 1980; 137: 327.

42. Ranney B: Endometriosis: IV. Herediatry tendency. Obstet Gynaecol 1971; 37: 734.

43. Sarraun M. Reezazadeh: Endometriosis in diagnostic laparoscopy in Isfahan fran. Jnt J Gynaecol Obstet 1986; 24: 117-19.

44. Lloyd FP: Endometriosis in Negro women. Am J Obstet Gynaecol 1964; 89: 468.

45. Minazawa K: Incidence of endometriosis among Japanese women. Obstet Gynaecol 1976; 48: 407.

46. Jones HW, Jr, Jones GK: Novak's text book of gynaecology 10th ed, Baltimore, Williams and wilkins 1981; pp.625.

47. Aleem M and Bashir A: Endometriosis and diagnostic laparoscopy. Specialist 1995; 11: 103-107.

48. APGO Educational Series on Women's Health Issues. Diagnosis & Management of Endometriosis: Pathophysiology to Practice 1-30.

49. Adamson GD, Kennedy S, Hummelshoj L. Creating solutions in endometriosis: global collaboration through the World Endometriosis Research Foundation. *J Endometriosis.* 2010;2(1):3-6.

50. Yeung P, Sinervo K, Winer W, Albee RB. Complete laparoscopic excision of endometriosis in teenagers: is postoperative hormonal suppression necessary? *Fertil Steril.* 2011; 95(6):1909-1912.

51. Kapoor D. Endometriosis. http://emedicine. medscape.com/article/271899-overview. Accessed June 23, 2012.

52. Koninckx PR. Epidemiology of endometriosis. www.gyns u rge ry.org/ o l s /pdf /030101_ Epidemiology%20of%20endometriosis.pdf. Accessed March 13 23, 2014.

53. Kokcu A. Relationship between endometriosis and cancer from current perspective. Arch Gynecol Obstet. 2011;284(6)1473-1479.

54. Mcleod BS, Retzloff MG. Epidemiology of endometriosis: an assessment of risk factors. Clin Obstet Gynecol. 2010;53(2):389-396.

55. Murphy AA. Clinical aspects of endometriosis. Ann N Y Acad Sci. 2002;955:1-10; discussion 34-6; 396-406.

56. Treloar SA, Bell TA, Nagle CM, Purdie DM, Green AC. Early menstrual characteristics associated with subsequent diagnosis of endometriosis. Am J Obstet Gynecol. 2010;202:534.e1-6.

57. Parazzini F, Ferraroni M, Fedele L, et al. Pelvic endometriosis: reproductive and menstrual risk factors at different stages in Lombardy, northern Italy. J Epidemiol Community Health. 1995; 49:61-64.

58. Matalliotakis IM, Arici A, Cakmak H, Goumenou AG, Koumantakis G, Mahutte NG. Familial aggregation of endometriosis in the Yale Series. Archives of Gynecology and Obstetrics. 2008;278(6):507-511.

59. Rier SE, Turner WE, Martin DC, Morris R, Lucier GW, Clark GC. Serum levels of TCDD and dioxin-like chemicals in Rhesus monkeys chronically exposed to dioxin: correlation of increased serum PCB levels with endometriosis. Toxicol Sci. 2001;59:147-159.

60. Giudice L, Evers JLH, Healy DL. Endometriosis: Science and Practice. Chichester, West Sussex: Wiley-Blackwell; 2012.

61. Matsuzaka Y, Kikuti YY, Goya K, et al. Lack of an association human dioxin detoxification gene polymorphisms with endometriosis in Japanese women: results of a pilot study. *Environ Health Prev Med.* Epub 1 May 2012.

62. Parazzini F, Cipriani S, Bianchi S, Gotsch F, Zanconato G, Fedele L. Risk factors for deep endometriosis: a comparison with pelvic and ovarian endometriosis. *Fertil Steril.* 2008; 90(1)174-179.

63. Vercellini P, Buggio L, Somigliana E, Barbara G, Vigano P, Fedele L. Attractiveness of women with rectovaginal endometriosis: a case-

control study. *Fertil Steril*. 2013;99(1):212-218. Epub 15 September 2012.

3 PATHOGENESIS OF ENDOMETRIOSIS

While the precise cause of endometriosis still remains unknown and is
the subject of debate, many theories have been promulgated to
comprehend better and elucidate its pathogenesis .These concepts
admittedly do not necessarily exclude each other. Furthermore no one
theory can explicate all cases of endometriosis [1], however the concept
of the aetiopathognesis seems flawed with the rapid surge of emerging
molecular and proteomic profiles of diseases. It is more than gratifying
to witness a revolution modifying influence on our current appreciation
of the pathophysiology and etiology of endometriosis.

Theories of Pathogenesis

The pathogenesis of endometriosis has been debated and most

theories fall into two broad divisions (1) Development in situ by metaplasia or (2) development as a consequence of the dissemination of endometrium [2]. The first widely considered theory of histogenesis was coelomic metaplasia; ovarian and Müllerian ducts are derived from coelomic mesothelium and it is proposed that the germinal epithelium of the ovary is responsible for endometriosis in this site [3]. This accounts for ovarian endometriosis. Endometriosis in the pelvis and peritoneum are considered to have developed from in situ metaplasia of the serosal mesothelium. However flaws in this theory exist, endometriosis has developed in women without endometrium (congenital absence of the uterus), also if coelomic metaplasia occurs in the peritoneum endometriosis would be found in men. Finally endometriosis should only then occur in sites with coelomic membranes – endometriosis has been found in every site in the body with exception of the spleen.

Sampson (1922& 1927) [4-5] initiated the theory of retrograde menstruation in 1927, in which he proposed that menstrual effluent contained viable endometrial cells that could be transplanted to ectopic sites. Retrograde menstruation is an event seen commonly in women [6], questioned why a physiological event should frequently give rise to pathology – and yet there has been no satisfactory explanation. Other researchers [7] proved that menstrual effluent did contain viable endometrial cells by culturing tissue fragments of endometrium. In support of this theory viable endometrial cells have been found in menstrual effluent and in the peritoneal fluid, endometrium can be implanted experimentally and grown within the peritoneal cavity and thirdly the fact that all women have some degree of retrograde menstruation. Dissemination of endometrial cells through lymphatic or vascular channels may account for the finding of endometriosis at sites distant from the pelvis.

Cases of endometriosis have been documented in episiotomy and laparotomy scars following gynaecological procedures and caesarean section. Such observations suggest that ectopic endometrium can be induced iatrogenically by mechanical transplantation [8].

Since Dr. Sampson first coined the term "endometriosis" in 1921 [4-5], extensive research on pathogenesis has been carried out. Despite progress, however, no single theory has proven sufficient to explain pathogenesis satisfactorily; current concepts hold that multifactorial immune, hormonal, genetic, environmental, and anatomic factors may be responsible.

According to Sampson's theory of retrograde menstruation, during a woman's menstrual flow, some of the endometrial efflux exits the uterus via the fallopian tubes and adheres to the peritoneal surface which it invades to produce endometriosis. While most women may have some retrograde menstrual flow, normally their immune system clears the debris thwarting implantation and occurrence of endometriosis,

Nevertheless, in some patients, misplaced endometrial tissue by retrograde menstruation may entrench to establish as endometriosis. Some of the possible causes that may predispose to the genesis of endometriosis include hereditary factors, toxins, or a compromised immune system. The failure of Sampson's theory to elucidate all instances of endometriosis implies that other factors such as genetic or immune differences have to be considered to explicate as to why many women with retrograde menstruation do not have endometriosis. In this context it is pertinent to quote one study that casts doubt on Sampson's theory based on finding of significant biochemical differences between endometriotic lesions and transplanted ectopic tissue [9] .

Retrograde menstruation is a fairly common physiologic event .But retrograde menstruation fails to adequately elucidate the extrauterine implantation of endometrial tissue. Diagnostic laparoscopy in the perimenstrual period shows that as many as 90% of women with patent fallopian tubes have bloody peritoneal fluid. However, the increase in risk of endometriosis is associated with conditions that augment the rate of retrograde menstruation, such as congenital outflow tract obstructions. This theory is supported by various animal experiments and clinical observations support this theory [9-12].

In an attempt to verify the Samson hypothesis Thomas et al 1995 [13], conducted experiment using baboons to determine the outcome of intrapelvic injection of menstrual versus luteal endometrium on the incidence, peritoneal involvement, and stage of endometriosis. concluded that Intrapelvic injection of menstrual endometrium can induce peritoneal endometriosis and provides experimental proof favouring the Sampson hypothesis.

It was postulated that when faulty endometrium with low levels of aberrant aromatase expression reaches the pelvic peritoneum by retrograde menstruation, it excites an inflammatory response that rapidly enhances local aromatase activity (i.e., estrogen formation) induced directly or indirectly by PGs and cytokines. The retrograde flow of menstrual blood via the fallopian tubes favours internal infection or inflammation of coelomic epithelial lining leading to conversion of some peritoneal cells into endometrial cells These ectopic foci respond to cyclic hormonal fluctuations in a manner akin to intrauterine endometrium, with proliferation, secretory activity, and cyclical sloughing of menstrual products.The products of this activity, coupled with the concerted and cyclic release of cytokines and prostaglandins, induces an altered inflammatory response characterized by neovascularization and fibrosis formation. Some investigators have been able to demonstrate abnormal T- and B-cell function, abnormal complement deposition, and altered interleukin (IL)-6 production in women with endometriosis

According to Seli E and Berkkanoglu Arici AM [1] the retrograde menstruation theory is commonly accepted. Retrograde menstruation occurs in 76% to 90% of women. The much reduced occurrence of endometriosis implies that there are additional factors that predispose to endometriosis. Endometriosis is linked with alterations in both cell-mediated and humoral immunity. Impaired natural killer cell activity leading to inadequate elimination of refluxed menstrual debris may play a role in the development of endometriotic implants. Furthermore, even though the peritoneal fluid of women with endometriosis contains augmented numbers of immune cells, these appear to assist rather than hinder the formation of endometriosis. Macrophages whose function is to clear endometrial cells from the peritoneal cavity seem to enhance their proliferation by secreting growth factors and cytokines. Although it is uncertain whether these immunologic changes provoke endometriosis or are a result of its presence, they appear to play an important role in allowing endometriosis implants to persist and progress and contribute to the development of associated infertility and pelvic pain. Danazol and gonadotropin-releasing hormone (GnRH) agonists have immunomodulatory effects are commonly used for the medical therapy of endometriosis. These drugs appear to down-regulate cellular and humoral immune responses connected with their effect on endometriotic implants [1].

Coelomic Metaplasia: Meyer's theory of coelomic metaplasia is entrenched in the concept that during embryogenesis, the coelomic epithelium with multipotent cells, lining the whole pelvic cavity can become transformed into endometriotic tissue; with maturation, these cells differentiate into specific organs or tissue. Nevertheless it is implicit that these differentiated cells can become "dedifferentiated", and result in   a new kind of tissue or organ This phenomenon is illustrated by the dedifferentiation of the cells that envelop the ovaries, to become endometrial cells.. Thus, these transformed endometrial cells on the ovary are subject to cyclic changes with menstruation, corresponding to its normal complement in the uterus. While the implantation and the metaplasia theories illustrate the mechanism of the initiation of endometriotic lesions, they do not explain the diverse clinical profile of endometriosis.

The metaplasia theory implies that under different influences, coelomic tissue could be transformed into endometrium. However, there has been no documented direct proof of the genesis of endometrial stroma at the conclusion of the metaplastic process. Furthermore this theory signifies that ectopic endometrium arises in situ from local tissues, including germinal epithelium of the ovary and remnants of the Müllerian and Wolffian ducts. Furthermore this theory implies that the origin of peritoneal endometriosis is from in situ metaplasia of totipotent mesothelial serosal cells. The predominance of endometriosis in females and hardly occurs in males, casts shadow of doubt on the conception of metaplasia to explain endometriosis.

Inflammation possibly triggers the change of one type of cell to the other [14]. At this juncture it is pertinent to delve further on the role of inflammation. Numerous cytokines including interleukin (IL)-1, 6, 8, 10, tumor necrosis factor (TNF)-alpha, and vascular endothelial growth factor (VEGF) were reported to be increased in the peritoneal fluid (PF) of women with endometriosis. Those cytokines may be concerned with macrophage activation, involved in inflammatory change and enhanced angiogenesis. Nevertheless reduced expression of some cytokines such as IL-2, and interferon (IFN)-gamma.was also found... They signify disturbed T- and natural killer (NK)-cell function. Endometriotic implants generate some factors, such as matrix metalloproteinases (MMPs), and Bcl-2, and impact their capacity to lodge in the peritoneum.Peritoneal cytokines, originating from mesothelial cells, leukocytes and ectopic endometrial cells, interact locally and systemically in women with endometriosis.

Yet another facet worth considering is the vital role of p38 mitogen-activated protein kinase (MAPK) in the process of inflammation is well recognized. Inflammation is conceived as an etiological factor for endometriosis Osamu Yoshino, et al 2006 [15], assessed in BALB/c mice, the outcome of FR 167653,(a p38 MAPK inhibitor), on the genesis of endometriosis. The estradiol-treated ovariectomized Balb/c mice representing endometriosis model, were injected intraperitoneally with small pieces of endometrial tissues of the syngenic donor mice. The animals were injected with either 30 mg/kg FR 167653 or only vehicle (control) s.c. twice a day, starting 2 days previous to endometrial injection. At the end of three weeks, the examination of peritoneal fluids and the induced endometriotic lesions.showed that the weight of all the endometriotic lesions per mouse and the levels of interleukin-6 and monocyte chemoattractant protein-1 in the peritoneal fluid were notably lesser in the FR 167653-treated mice relative to that in the control mice. These observations imply the inhibitory effect of FR 167653 on the development of endometriosis probably by suppressed peritoneal inflammation [15].

Both Sampson retrograde menstruation, and implantation and the metaplasia theory focus upon the implantation/metaplasia of cells, and thus on subtle lesions, i.e. small initial lesions, which will subsequently grow and develop to more severe disease. These theories are attractive because of the abundance of data demonstrating retrograde menstruation as a frequent phenomenon occurring almost in all women, the presence in peritoneal fluid of viable endometrial cells, which have the capacity to implant, to grow and to infiltrate superficially. According to this view, the development into a more severe condition may be influenced by a decreased cellular immunity, a lower NK cell activity, peritoneal fluid cytokines and growth factors, or low peritoneal fluid steroid concentrations in the luteal phase [16].

These theories are attractive since each step in the pathophysiology has been documented. It is important to recognize that this theory, cannot explain why progression occurs in some women only. Fundamentally this theory holds that progression of endometriosis once established is unavoidable, albeit at a different speed and to a different stage according to modulating factors. Essentially, this theory considers endometriosis as normal endometrial cells which behave abnormally, because of the abnormal environment, i.e. the peritoneal milieu. This is however, not supported by all [16-17]. The key event in the process is implantation or metaplasia, which thus has been the subject of many investigations, and the early subtle lesions become very important.

The endometriotic disease theory considers retrograde menstruation, viable endometrial cells in peritoneal fluid, and occasional implantation of some of these cells a normal physiological phenomenon. These non-implanted and implanted cells are normally removed by the defense mechanisms of the body such as macrophages [18].

Attachment and implantation is favourized when the mesothelial layer is damaged by trauma, infection or even by low grade inflammation, e.g. irritation caused by CO_2 pneumoperitoneum, or by abundant retrograde menstruation. It also seems logical that attachment and implantation must occur more frequently when more viable cells are present in peritoneal fluid. Although these cells can temporarily grow and develop depending upon the environment, their ultimate fate when left alone will be their spontaneous disappearance. This can result in some fibrotic or scar tissue as the remnant of local inflammation, containing eventually some endometrial cells, shielded from the blood stream and immunocompetent cells comparable to the bacteria in an abscess [16,18].

The much lower prevalence of endometriosis implies that other factors determine propensity to endometriosis Notwithstanding this theory has its pros and cons An observation that endorses this theory is the increased incidence of endometriosis in women with augmented retrograde menstruation as they menstruate more frequently or have a congenitally absent cervix. Retrograde menstruation via the fallopian tubes into the peritoneal cavity is a very frequent physiologic occurrence in all menstruating women with patent tubes. Although approximately 90% of women may have some degree of retrograde menstruation not all develop endometriosis [19]. This has engendered another hypothesis that women with endometriosis have reduced immunological clearance of misplaced endometrial cells within the peritoneal cavity.

Some of the possible causes that may predispose to the genesis of endometriosis include hereditary factors, toxins, or a compromised immune system. The downside of this theory is its failure to elucidate all instances of endometriosis; hence this implies that other factors such as genetic or immune differences have to be hypothesized to explain as to why many women with retrograde menstruation do not have endometriosis. In this context it is pertinent to quote one study that casts doubt on Sampson's theory based on finding of significant biochemical differences between endometriotic lesions and transplanted ectopic tissue.

Role of Estrogens:

Endometriosis being an estrogen-dependent condition is seen primarily during the reproductive years. In experimental models, estrogen is necessary to induce or maintain endometriosis. Medical therapy is often targeted at lowering estrogen levels to contain the disease. Additionally, research on aromatase, an estrogen-synthesizing enzyme, has provided evidence for the continuation of endometriosis after menopause and hysterectomy.

Endometriosis, as already stated earlier develops mostly in women of reproductive age and regresses after menopause or ovariectomy, signifying that the growth is estrogen-dependent [20].

In experimental models, estrogen is necessary to induce or maintain endometriosis. Obviously medical therapy is often intended to reduce estrogen levels to manage the disease. Additionally, the current research focus on aromatase, an estrogen-synthesizing enzyme, has amply proved the pathogenesis of endometriosis after menopause and hysterectomy. Aromatase P450 (P450arom), the key enzyme for biosynthesis of estrogen, is a vital hormone for the genesis and development of endometriosis. No obvious aromatase activity is present in normal endometrium, hence estrogen is not locally formed in endometrium. On the contrary endometriotic tissue, is rich with extremely elevated levels of aromatase [21], which stimulates substantial production of estrogen. In addition prostaglandin, an important mediator of inflammation appreciably induces aromatase activity producing in turn local estrogen in this tissue. Estrogen also stimulates cyclo-oxygenase-2 augmenting the formation of prostaglandin E_2 in endometriosis [21].

Serdar E. Bulun et al 2004 [21], have demonstrated an "intracrine" effect of estrogen in uterine leiomyomas and endometriosis: Estrogen produced by aromatase activity in the cytoplasm of leiomyoma smooth muscle cells or endometriotic stromal cells can affect by readily binding to its nuclear receptor within the same cell [22-24].

In contrast, normal endometrium and myometrium, are deficient in aromatase expression [23-24]. Aromatase catalyzes the conversion of androstenedione and testosterone to estrone and estradiol. The gene that encodes this enzyme is articulated in numerous human tissue cells including ovarian granulosa cells, adipose tissue, skin, fibroblasts, and the brain. As is well known in woman of reproductive-age the ovary is the principal organ for estrogen biosynthesis, and this takes place in a cyclic fashion. Upon binding of follicle-stimulating hormone (FSH) to its G-protein-coupled receptor in the granulosa cell membrane, intracellular cyclic adenosine monophosphate (cAMP) levels increase and enhance binding of two critical transcription factors [i.e., steroidogenic factor-1 (SF-1) and cAMP response element binding protein (CREB)], to the typically sited proximal promoter II of the aromatase gene [25-26]. This, in turn, activates aromatase expression and consequently estrogen secretion from the preovulatory follicle [26].

Alternatively, in postmenopausal women, estrogen formation occurs in the adipose tissue and skin [27-29]. Contrary to cAMP regulation of aromatase expression in the ovary, this is controlled mainly by cytokines [interleukin (IL)-6, IL-11, tumor necrosis factor alpha (TNFα)] and glucocorticoids via the alternative use of promoter I.4 in adipose tissue and skin fibroblasts [30]. The key substrate for aromatase in adipose tissue and skin is androstenedione from adrenals. In postmenopausal women, ~2% of circulating androstenedione is converted to estrone, which is further changed to estradiol in these peripheral tissues.

Extensive and intensive studies on aromatase expression in endometriosis [31-32], revealed exceedingly elevated levels of aromatase mRNA in extraovarian endometriotic implants and endometriomas. In addition endometriosis-derived stromal cells in culture incubated with a cAMP analog exhibited exceptionally high levels of aromatase activity [33] Further investigations on stimulators of aromatase activity via a cAMP-dependent pathway in endometriosis revealed that Prostaglandin E_2 (PGE_2) as the most powerful inducer of aromatase activity in endometriotic stromal cells [33]. mediated via the cAMP-inducing EP_2 receptor subtype Additionally, estrogen was found to enhance PGE_2 formation by stimulating cyclooxygenase type 2 (COX-2) enzyme in endometrial stromal cells in culture [34]. The establishment of constant local production of estrogen and prostaglandins (PGs), leads to the proliferative and inflammatory features of endometriosis Aromatase micro RNA was detected in the eutopic endometrial samples of women with moderate to severe endometriosis and absent in disease-free women albeit in much lesser quantities relative to endometriotic implants. This weak finding in the eutopic endometrium. may imply a genetic fault in women with endometriosis It is postulated by Serdar E. Bulunet al, that when faulty endometrium with low levels of aberrant aromatase expression reaches the pelvic peritoneum by retrograde menstruation, it excites an inflammatory response that rapidly enhances local aromatase activity (i.e., estrogen formation) induced directly or indirectly by PGs and cytokines [32]. The clinical relevance of aromatase expression is best appreciated if aromatase inhibitors could be of benefit in the treatment of endometriosis. In addition to aberrant aromatase expression other important factors in molecular mechanism may be involved in the pathogenesis of pelvic endometriosis ;these factors may include 1) abnormal expression of matrix metalloproteinases, tissue inhibitor of metalloproteinase-, 2) certain cytokines (IL-6, RANTES (regulated on activation, normal T cell expressed and secreted), and 3) epidermal growth factor [35-36]. Furthermore another proposal for the genesis of endometriosis has been suggested. That pinpoints to a flawed immune system that fails to eliminate peritoneal surfaces of the retrograde menstrual flow the development of endometriosis [37].

Undeniably the endometriotic lesions have estrogen receptors (ER) as well as aromatase, that catalyses the conversion of androgens to estrogens, signifying that local estrogen production may fuel the growth of lesions. It is notable that the expression patterns of ER and progesterone receptors in endometriotic lesions are different from those in the eutopic endometrium. Additionally estrogen metabolism, including the expression pattern of aromatase and the regulation of 17 beta-hydroxysteroid dehydrogenase type 2 (an enzyme responsible for the inactivation of estradiol to estrone), is changed in the eutopic endometrium of women with endometriosis, adenomyosis, and/or leiomyomas compared to that in the eutopic endometrium of normal women. Immunostaining for P450arom in endometrial biopsy specimens diagnosed these diseases with sensitivity and specificity of 91 and 100%, respectively. This is valuable in the clinical diagnosis of endometriosis. The polymorphisms in the ER-alpha gene, the CYP19 gene encoding aromatase, and several other genes are linked with the risk of endometriosis. Studies focusing on these will lead to better understanding of the etiopathogensis of endometriosis [38]. That estrogen has a vital role in the immune response in immune-mediated diseases hardly needs any reiteration. Estrogen receptors are expressed in a variety of immunocompetent cells, including CD4(+) and CD8(+) T cells and macrophages Based on a distinct profile of cytokine production, data accrued hitherto have shown modulatory effects for estrogen on the TH1-type and TH2-type cells, which signify two distinctly clear cut forms of the effector specific immune response. Recent evidence indicates that estrogens inhibit the production of TH1 proinflammatory cytokines, such as IL-12, TNF-alpha and IFN-gamma; on the contrary estrogens encourage the generation of TH2 anti-inflammatory cytokines, such as IL-10, IL-4, and TGF-beta.

Salem ML, 2004 [39], postulated that estrogen aggravates or suppresses inflammatory diseases mediated by skewing TH1-type to TH2-type response. This view conceptualizes a novel mechanism for the modulatory impact of estrogen on certain inflammatory diseases that can result in useful or unfavorable outcomes depending on the type of immune response involved.

Role of other hormones

While we have drawn our attention to estrogens and their role in endometriosis it is essential to focus on the role of other hormones in the pathogenesis of this disorder. It is known that the periodic expression of matrix metalloproteinases (MMPs) by human endometrium has been implicated to play a part in the invasive process essential to set up endometriosis. Progesterone can inhibit endometrial MMP-3 and MMP-7 expression and this requires the local action of $TGF\beta$ and may also be associated with the local generation of retinoic acid by stromal cells. A constant expression of several MMPs in endometriotic lesions has been reported, indicating a failure of progesterone or locally produced factors to suppress these enzymes. This leads us to focus on the therapeutic relevance of Progestins which are effective in endometriosis but , the precise mechanisms of their action still remain unresolved. The investigative studies of Verena Mönckedieck,et al 2009 [40], are worthy of mention. They throw light on the role of progesterone in endometriosis. They studied employing nude mice , the impact of different progestins on notable features of extracellular matrix degradation and angiogenesis implicated in the setting up and continuation of ectopic endometrial lesions. The study involved intraperitoneal transplantation of human endometrium into nude mice.

Following one week and four weeks of treatment with progesterone, dydrogesterone, or its metabolite dihydrodydrogesterone, respectively, they evaluated ectopic lesions for proliferation and apoptosis expression of estrogen receptor α, progesterone receptor-AB, the angiogenetic factors, cysteine-rich angiogenic inducer (CYR61), basic fibroblast growth factor (bFGF), vascular endothelial growth factor (VEGFA) and the matrix metalloproteinase (MMP)-2, -3, -7 and -9. In addition functional influence on angiogenesis was also assessed .Even though dydrogesterone appreciably reduced proliferation of endometrial stromal cells the end of four weeks, suppression of apoptosis was unrelated to progestins. While all progestins substantially reduced expression of MMP-2 and dydrogesterone reduced MMP-3. In the grafted endometrial tissue, progesterone and dihydrodydrogesterone, suppressed transcription of bFGF and VEGFA and CYR61 were suppressed by dihydrodydrogesterone and dydrogesterone. Microvessel density was slightly suppressed by progestins, while number of stabilized vessels increased. Thus, progestins control factors vital for the genesis and continuance of ectopic endometrial lesions [40].

It is of interest at this juncture to allude to the role of MMP and TIMP in mediating the survival and implantation of endometrial cells in the peritoneal fluid. Matrix metalloproteinases (MMPs) have play a part in the degradation and turnover of extracellular matrix proteins and their action is regulated by specific tissue inhibitors called tissue inhibitors of metalloproteinases (TIMPs). In a study comparing the concentrations of total and active MMP-9 in peritoneal fluid of 22 infertile men with mild or moderate endometriosis and those with those in a control group of 21.infertile patients it was found that the mean total concentrations of MMP-9 in the peritoneal fluid of patients with endometriosis was almost thrice higher (6.2 ± 1.8 ng/ml), compared to the concentration of 2.9 ± 2.6 ng/ml in the control group .There was no significant difference in the levels of active MMP-9 between the groups. The concentrations of TIMP-1, were appreciably lower in endometriotic peritoneal fluids than in peritoneal fluid of control women,(1.02 ± 0.21 ng/ml and 1.16 ± 0.18 ng/ml respectively. Neither was any correlation between stage of disease, steroid hormone concentration, MMP-9 (total and active) and TIMP-1 was found. Thus their findings imply that the disequilibrium between MMP-9 and TIMP-1 in peritoneal fluid of women with endometriosis may play a significant role in the pathogenesis of the disease [41]. On reaching the peritoneal cavity, the survival and implantation of endometrial cells seem to be mediated by abnormal MMP and TIMP expression, altered immune milieu, aberrant local aromatase activity, and genetic and environmental factors [42].

Müllerianosis: Another theory proposes that cells with the potential to differentiate into endometrial cells are laid down in paths that during embryonic development and organogenesis. These tracts follow the Mullerian tract as it moves caudally at 8–10 weeks of embryonic life.

Primitive endometrial cells become displaced from the migrating uterus and act like <u>stem cells</u>. This theory is supported by foetal autopsy. Müllerianosis is exactly the condition of "developmentally misplaced endometrial tissue," [43].

Batt RE, et al 2007 [43], defined it as an organoid structure of embryonic descent a choristoma made up of müllerian rests--normal endometrium, normal endosalpinx, and normal endocervix--singly or in combination, included within other normal organs during organogenesis.. Histologically, endometrial-müllerianosis and endometriosis both comprise endometrial glands and stroma, Notwithstanding both these conditions have different pathogenesis. Batt RE, et al 1990 [44] suggested that müllerianosis is a distinctive form of endometriosis, which differs in its pathogenesis from all forms of transplantation endometriosis be it of lymphatic, hematogenous, transtubal, or iatrogenic origin; it is also separate from endometriosis of coelomic metaplasia [44].

Müllerianosis' has borad connotation to in clue collection of epithelial and mesenchymal 'metaplasias' and proliferations that are usual in the female peritoneal cavity, commonly around the pelvic viscera and particularly the ovaries. In many ways, their morphological features identical to their cellular analogues lining or forming the müllerian duct derivatives, such as endosalpinx (the fallopian tube mucosal lining), endometrium,and smooth muscle It is pertinent to refer to Sampson's classification of misplaced endometrial or müllerian tissue into "four or possibly five groups, on the basis of the manner this tissue deposited at ectopic site. Sampson [5] classified aberrant or misplaced endometrial tissue on the grounds of its pathogenesis: 1) direct or primary endometriosis [adenomyosis]; an analogous form occurs in the wall of the fallopian tube from its mucosal incursion [endosalpingiosis]; 2) peritoneal or implantation endometriosis; 3) transplantation endometriosis; 4) metastatic endometriosis; and 5) developmentally misplaced endometrial tissue [4-5].

In vitro study of secretion profile of IL and growth factors (VEGF, IGF-I, TGFbeta) by endometrial tissues and endometrioid heterotopies in patients with external genital endometriosis revealed enhanced production of IL-1beta, IL-2, IL-6, and VEGF in the endometrium in severe external genital endometriosis, and decreased secretion of TGFbeta; but just the opposite profile was seen in endometrioid foci. In all probability local cytokine imbalance and enhanced proliferative activity of endometrial cells are implicated in the pathogenesis of endometrioid foci. Other than the role of interleukins and growth factors referred to above in the genesis of endometriosis the importance of c-myc protooncogene and its polypeptide product significant regulator of cell proliferation and differentiation in the pathogenesis of endometriosis.was explored.It is assumed ovarian steroids promote growth of different uterine cell types through altered expression of the c-myc gene. With the aim to verify this assumption whether c-myc expression may also be involved in the genesis and growth of endometriosis, Schenken RS, et al 1991 [45], evaluated c-myc expression in eutopic and ectopic endometrial tissue from women undergoing surgery for endometriosis. Immunocytochemical studies revealed positive staining for c-myc protein in both glandular cytoplasm and nuclei and only stromal cell nuclei, in both eutopic and ectopic endometrium. This finding impies that c-myc expression may be a key controller of cell proliferation in endometriotic tissue.

Angiogenesis

While various theories attempt to elucidate the occurrence of extrauterine endometrial tissue, none of them can either satisfactorily explain all disease locations and appearances or the manner these fragments establish into endometriotic lesions [46]. It is relevant at this juncture to allude the release of VEGF along with IL 6810 and TNF which are all increased in peritoneal fluid of women with endometriosis [14].

Obviously angiogenesis is possibly with VEGF. New vessel formation has long been recognized as a feature of endometriosis, often clearly visible at laparoscopy. Recent work has focused on identifying the role of vascularization in the pathogenesis of endometriosis, by allowing lesions to establish and grow [46].

This theory is further fortified by laboratory documentation of this conversion. In vitro experimental model of endometriosis employing human ovarian surface epithelial cells supports the metaplastic origin of endometriotic lesions from the ovarian surface epithelium. The model of Matsuura K, et al [47], entailimg coculture of both ovarian surface epithelium and ovarian stromal cells with 17beta estradiol revealed that the ovarian surface epithelium cells produced a luminal structure, encircled by endometrial stromal cells with an epithelial mesenchymal structure.That endometriosis may result from a sequential transformation from the adjacent mesothelial cells is further confirmed by immunopositivity of epithelial membrane antigen and cytokeratin in the glandular cells and cilia, as well as in the microvilli. coupled with the EM findings of tight junctions on cell surfaces [47].

The autoimmune theory of endometriosis

Before we go to specific issue of the autoimmune etiology of endometriosis it will useful to recapitulate briefly the concept of autoimmune diseases. Majority of autoimmune diseases occur in women, and these are most commonly in reproductive age group. The reasons for this higher gender predominance are still unclear, some autoimmune diseases occur more often in postmenopausal women. It is of interest to note that while in some cases pregnancy has an ameliorating influence on this disease while in others it is aggravated by pregnancy.There may exacerbations of the illness following delivery.

As for its etiology it is possibly multifactorial involving genetics, environmental and hormonal factors. The disease has a genetic basis as it is seen as clusters in certain families. Different members of a family can have varying types of autoimmune diseases.

The pathogenesis of autoimmune diseases and autoimmune reactions

Autoimmune reactions can be triggered in several ways:

- A substance in the body that is normally strictly contained in a specific area (and thus is hidden from the immune system) is released into the general circulation. For example, the fluid in the eyeball is normally contained within the eyeball's chambers. If a blow to the eye releases this fluid into the bloodstream, the immune system may react against it.

- A normal body substance is altered. For example, viruses, drugs, sunlight, or radiation may change a protein's structure in a way that makes it seem foreign.

- The immune system responds to a foreign substance that is similar in appearance to a natural body substance and inadvertently targets the body substance as well as the foreign substance.

Something malfunctions in the cells that control antibody production. For example, cancerous B lymphocytes may produce abnormal antibodies that attack red blood cells

Having briefly dealt with the fringe of the problem of broad aspect of autoimmune diseases we shall consider some of the current concepts with regards to autoimmune nature of endometriosis.

The intriguing question is endometriosis an autoimmune aiseases question apart we shall consider some of the known aspects of the disease. The link between antiendometrial anibodies and endometriosis will be touched upon here. An important factor in the pathogenesis and progression of endometriosis could be attributed to, a failure in the immune system tolerance to self-antigens, resulting in an autoimmune condition. The detection of antiendometrial antibodies both in peritoneal fluid and serum of women with endometriosis is an undeniable proof for this autoimmune phenomenon. The spectrum of autoimmune alterations comprises a decrease in NK activity, increased generation of proinflammatory cytokines, and enhanced angiogenic activity. Additionally the striking similarity between the immunological profile in experimentally induced endometriosis in a Wistar rat model and those seen in human, is noteworthy [48].

Apart from antiendometrial antibodies other antibodies such as antinuclear antibody.and lupus anticoagfulant antibody have been found in endometriosis patients Besides immunoglobulin IgG autroantibodies,and IgM autoantibodies have also been found in patients with endometriosis. Among IgG autoantibodies, those to phospholipids were most common, followed in order of frequency by antibodies to histones and nucleotides. The incidence of IgM autoantibodies was reversed, with antinucleotides appearing most frequently and antiphospholipids least frequently. These findings imply that endometriosis is linked with abnormal polyclonal B cell activation, a typical feature of autoimmune disease. This argument is further fortified by the elevated levels immunoglobulin (principally IgG) in patients with endometriosis, and more so in lupus anticoagulant-positive than lupus anticoagulant-negative endometriosis patients.

Among 59 laparoscopically staged endometriosis patients, 28.8% tested positive for antinuclear antibody. Of 44 patients, 45.5% were lupus anticoagulant positive (greater than 1.3) and 20.5% were within a borderline range (1.2-1.3). Antinuclear antibody positivity was inversely related to stage of disease (P = .009); lupus anticoagulant positivity exhibited a similar trend, but did not reach statistical significance. Of 31 endometriosis patients, 64.5% exhibited immunoglobulin G (IgG) autoantibodies and 45.2% demonstrated IgM autoantibodies to at least one of 16 antigens investigated. Among IgG autoantibodies, those to phospholipids were most frequently detected, followed in order of frequency by antibodies to histones and nucleotides. The incidence of

IgM autoantibodies was inverted, with antinucleotides appearing most frequently and antiphospholipids least frequently. A strong correlation was noted between the presence of lupus anticoagulant and antinuclear antibody with both IgG and IgM autoantibodies. These observations suggest that endometriosis is associated with abnormal polyclonal B cell activation, a typical feature of autoimmune disease. The elevated immunoglobulin levels (particularly IgG) in patients with endometriosis, further support this contention and more so in lupus anticoagulant-positive than lupus anticoagulant-negative endometriosis patients

The following may further illustrate the relevance of the theory of autoimmune nature of endometriosis. In addition it is to be appreciated that a mosaic of antibodies has added to the myriad complexities of the undeniably complicated disease.Just to illustrate briefly the type of antibodies we have cited some of the following.

In investigating immunoglobulins IgG, IgA and IgM against endometrial antigens in patients with endometriosis and fertile controls were tested (Ig)G, IgA, or IgM in endometrium, serum, and peritoneal fluid (PF) of the patients and controls using Western blot analysis. Mathur S,et al 1990 [49], observed the presence of endogenous IgG in 78% of the endometria or endometriosis implants from the patients and 22% of the endometria from the controls and endometrial IgA and IgM were detectable in few controls and patients. Further it was observed that

IgG in the serum and/or PF of patients with endometriosis was specifically aimed at only certain antigens (i.e.with molecular weights of 34, 42, 82, 94, 110, 120, and 140 kd) found in the patients' endometrium or endometriosis implants. IgA and IgM in the serum or PF of the patients and controls were nonspecific in their reactivity. Endometrial antigens in endometrium or endometriotic implants of patients with endometriosis, and drawing IgG responses, may be applicable to and consistent with autoimmunity in endometriosis [49].

The identification of endometrial antigens provoking autoimmunity would establish an antibody assay which would serve both as a non-invasive diagnostic test as well as a monitoring aid in clinical assessment of endometriosis. With this objective Pillai S etal, [50], performed systematic study of Forty-six women with endometriosis, 4 women with uterine leiomyomata, 4 with pelvic adhesions, 3 with repeat Cesarean sections (conditions that coexist with or predispose to endometriosis) and 46 controls. The investigations comprising Two-dimensional gel electrophoresis of endometrial extracts, Western blot analysis, passive hemagglutination and enzyme-linked immunosorbent assay (ELISA), amino acid sequencing and molecular studies on chosen antigens revealed that endometriosis patients had appreciable IgG antibodies to two endometrial antigens transferrin and alpha 2-HS-glycoprotein. The highlight of this study is the diagnostic value of an antibody assay using these antigens for diagnosing endometriosis [50].

Prompted by the objective to explore the presence and clinical correlation of serum autoantibodies to carbonic anhydrase (CA) in women with and without endometriosis. D'Cruz OJ,et al 1996 [51], tested sera of 319 patients with laproscopically diagnosed pelvic endomertiosis in varying stages ,100 with other gynecologic problems and 100 control women. Positive sera also were systematically tested for antiendometrial antibodies and antinuclear antibodies (ANA) antibodies to single-stranded (ss) and double-stranded (ds) DNA, and extractable nuclear antigens (Sm, nRNP, Ro, and La). The study revealed that; a)a subgroup of patients with endometriosis had autoantibodies to native and linear epitopes of the CA protein, b) occurrence of anti-CA antibodies was linked with antiendometrial antibodies and ANA.and c) Anti-CA antibodies were allied with a higher prognostic value of the disease when all patient subgroups were considered together [51].

Another investigative study of the connection of rheumatoid arthritis-associated single nucleotide polymorphisms in endometriosis.merits mentioned. It revealed an association of CCL21 (rs2812378) and HLA-DRB1 (rs660895) with moderate to severe endometriosis [52].

It is suggested that the pathogenesis of endometriosis involves abnormal immunologic mechanism Fc receptor-like 3 gene (FCRL3) has been projected as a novel autoimmune predisposing factor. Prompted by hypothesis of a probable association between endometriosis, infertility and FCRL3 polymorphisms. The authors conducted a case-control study comprising 170 women with endometriosis-related infertility, 91 women with idiopathic infertility and 166 controls. Using TaqMan PCR, they performed detection of FCRL3 polymorphisms (-169C/T, -110G/A, +358C/G and +1381A/G). Systematic statistrical analysis of the single-marker analysis revealed that FCRL3-169C/T was appreciably coupled with endometriosis (p=0.004), irrespective of the stage of the disease, p=0.011 and p=0.035, respectively [52].

Another theory has it that the normal occurrence of endometrial reflux in the fallopian tubes during menstruation may, in some circumstances, surmount local defense mechanisms, implant, and proliferate. Nevertheless, the presence of endometriosis in sites far removed from pelvic organs led to the quest for other theories such as genetic background, embryonic rest theory and stem cell dysfunction: The stem cell theory does not only substantiate the findings of endometriosis at distant sites away from the peritoneal cavity,but also elucidates resistance to some treatments, and the infrequently occurs even after hysterectomy. Recently, it was demonstrated that bone marrow–derived (mesenchymal) stem cells could lead to expression of endometriosis in a mouse model [53].

Another study demonstrated how endometriosis was initiated from stem cells, in a mouse model whose uterus was removed so that endometriosis could not originate from endometrial cells (either through retrograde menstruation, or hematogenous or lymphatic dissemination). In their experimental model, stem cells populated endometriotic implants, leading to disease progression. They observed the presence of stem cells in nearly every one of the organs of the body including the peritoneal cavity and uterus.

With a view to confirm the proposition of the existence of a likely endometriosis inducing factor(s) (EIF) in the blood of women with endometriosis. Rasheed K,et al [53], investigated fifteen women of each three different degrees of endometriosis and fifteen women without endometriosis as a control group. The women sera were co-cultured with mesenchymal stem cells (MSCs) which were followed up weekly to look for morphological changes and to detect Annexin 1 marker and ß-actin gene by reverse transcriptase polymerase chain reaction. MSCs cultured with sera of all cases regardless of the severity of endometriosis, exhibited morphological alterations resembling endometrial like cells and glands- by the 4th week in 60%, 60% & 100% respectively. These cells were seen from the first week in women with moderate and severe types (20% for each group). There proportion of the transformation into endometrial like cells augmented in an ascending order among the three groups where it was 30±25.8%, 45±29.9% and 75±37.9% respectively. Additionally number of endometrial like cells detected weekly ,are found increasing with the severity of disease is. There was no change in any of the the cultures of serum of the control group Besides,with progressive differentiation the density of stem cells decreased substantially.and the differentiated cells expressed the Annexin-1 marker.: These data evidently support that serum of women with endometriosis has a factor(s) that induces the alteration of the MSCs into endometrial like cells and glands in vitro. This finding not only substantiate a new theory for the etiology of endometriosis but also may . have a potential implication on the therapy of this debilitating condition [53].

Endometriosis is tacitly supposed to be a progressive disease, with inevitable growth and development of lesions once the disease has set in According to a novel concept the transition of endometriosis to endometriotic disease is regarded as identical to the origin and evolution of a benign tumour. This conception obviously implicates cellular alterations such as mutations. According to this theory endometriosis develops from endometriotic cells that have 'escaped' the influence of protective and regulatory factors in the peritoneal fluid [18].

In this context it is pertinent to allude to the the possible role of the immune system which can recognize and eliminate altered or misplaced autologous cells such as ectopic endometrial cells. This mechanism may operate in most women, preventing the development of endometriosis. Functional alterations of cells of the immune system in women with endometriosis have been observed; these functional changes affect monocytes/macrophages, natural killer cells, cytotoxic T-lymphocytes and B cells. In the light of these observations in women with endometriosis it is probable that these changes involve diminished surveillance, recognition and obliteration of the ectopic endometrial cells and potential facilitation of their implantation and development of endometriosis. Peripheral blood monocytes (PBM) and peritoneal macrophages (PM) may play a key role in this regard, and may control function of other immune cells. Dmowski WP et al 1996 [54], have shown that in normal fertile women without endometriosis, PBM and PM repress endometrial cell proliferation in vitro. In endometriosis, PBM stimulate and PM inhibit endometrial cell proliferation and the cytotoxic effect of PM is inversely correlated with the stage of the disease. The decrease in PM cytotoxic function is controlled by prostaglandin synthesis. In infertile women without endometriosis, the effects of PM and PBM are variable. In about a third of patients, the effects of PM and PBM suggest subclinical endometriosis; in the remaining patients the effects of PM and PBM are similar to those of fertile controls. It is noteworthy that endometrial cells in women with endometriosis are more sensitive to the stimulatory effect of PBM, and more resistant to the cytotoxicity of the immune cells [54].

At this juncture it seems relevant to make reference also to the association of p53 polymorphisms with endometriosis impelled by the aim of assessing the link between endometriosis and the p53 polymorphism . Chi Chen Chang,.et al 2002 [55], conducted a prospective study enrolling 118 women with and 140 without endometriosis. The former were grouped as those with moderate or severe endometriosis and the other without endometriosis. By Polymerase chain reaction p53 codon 72 polymorphisms (arginine homozygosity, heterozygosity, and proline homozygosity) was detected. The evaluation of relations between endometriosis and p53 polymorphisms observed that the distributions of diverse p53 polymorphisms differed remarkably between groups. The endometriosis group showed level of 10.2%, 66.9%, and 22.9% respectively arginine homozygotes, heterozygotes, and proline homozygotes and 30.7%, 50%, and 19.3% in the group without endometriosis. In addition to the findings of the association of endometriosis with p53 polymorphism.it was found that p53 arginine homozygotes have reduced risk for endometriosis while Heterozygotes and proline homozygotes are exposed to increased risk for endometriosis [55].

Further it is of interest to quote the observations of Vercellini P, et al 1994 on the analysis of p53 and ras gene mutations in endometriosis. Variceli et al 1994 [56], reported that no activating mutations in codons 12, 13 and 61 of ras genes nor inactivating mutations in exons 5-9 of the p53 tumor suppressor gene were detected by polymerase chain reaction and single-strand conformation polymorphism methods in either eutopic or ectopic endometrium from 10 women with severe endometriosis [56].

Molecular Aspects of Endometriosis:

Research also showed that exogeneous Annexin-1 can protect cells from necrosis induced by hydrogen peroxide [57]. Thus, increased Annexin-1 levels may inhibit the necrosis of refluxed endometrial cells and keep them viable, which is necessary for the development of endometriosis [58]. Annexin-1 functions as a substrate for the EGF receptor tyrosine kinase, which has a significant role in cell proliferation and differentiation [59]. Additionally, it holds phosphorylation sites for significant proliferative signaling molecules, including several signal transducing kinase associated hepatocyte growth factor receptor [60], and protein kinase C [61]. The overexpression of Annexin-1 may promote the proliferation of endometrial cells by modulating these signal transduction pathways [58].

The relation between Annexin-1 and the immune system and its expression in the peritoneal fluids possibly may render the peritoneal micromelieu conducive for implantation and growth of refluxed endometrial cells leading to endometriosis. Endometriosis , is known as a local pelvic inflammatory disorder.. It has been shown that macrophages in the peritoneal fluid participate dynamically in the start, upkeep and evolution of endometriosis [62]. Changes in T cell-mediated immunity take place in patients with endometriosis [61]. It has been shown that Annexin-1 has many functions attributed to it ;it controls activities of both the innate and adaptive immune cells such as macrophages and T lymphocytes,and regulates the phagocytic potential of macrophages and its production of TNF-α and IL-6., Annexin 1 derived peptides suppress antigen-driven cellular proliferation and cytokine production. Annexin-1 augments anti-CD3/CD28- mediated CD25 and CD69 expression, and increases the activation and proliferation of T cells in response to anti-CD3 plus anti-CD28 stimulation. Elevated levels of Annexin-1 in both endometrium and in peritoneal fluids may alter the components of the peritoneal fluids and the local immune microenvironment.Thus endometriosis may develop once a defective "disposal system" allows the implantation and growth of endometrial cells or fragments [60]. Thus, the overexpression of Annexin-1 in eutopic endometrium, and its presence in the peritoneal fluids of women with endometriosis, might increase the survival and proliferation of refluxed endometrial cells, and may also make the pelvic environment become "permissive" to their adherence and implantation.

Chun found from their study, expression of Annexin-1 protein mostly in endometrial glandular cells during the menstrual cycle, signifying that Annexin-1 may act on endometrial glandular and the stromal cells by autocrine or paracrine mechanisms, without significant change with the hormone levels. The actual mechanism of Annexin-1 on endometrial cells warrant further investigation [58].

Cytokines and endometriosis:

From an extensive review it was obvious that numerous cytokines including interleukin (IL)-1, 6, 8, 10, tumor necrosis factor (TNF)-α, and vascular endothelial growth factor (VEGF) were found enhanced in the peritoneal fluid (PF) of women with endometriosis. These cytokines are possibly concerned with in macrophage activation, inflammatory change and augmented angiogenesis. Nevertheless, some cytokines such as IL-2, and interferon (IFN)-γ.were less expressed. They signify the impaired T- and natural killer (NK)-cell function. Endometriotic implants generate some factors, e.g. matrix metalloproteinases (MMPs), Bcl-2, and upset their potential to implant into the peritoneum. There is, a local and systemic, interplay between cytokines and leucocytes and endometrial cells in women with endometriosis. Further studies about the specific role and interactions of these cytokines are warranted to enhance the understanding of endometriosis in order to develop newl therapies [14].

The TNF-alpha concentration in the peritoneal fluid considerably correlated with the menstrual cycle day (P < 0.01), with increasing concentration as the menstrual cycle progressed from the follicular to the luteal phase. On the other hand , IL-1 and IL-6 levels did not vary throughout the menstrual cycle. Increased TNF-alpha was found in patients with pelvic adhesions compared with those with normal pelvis; the concentration of TNF-alpha was highest in mild compared with severe adhesions, but IL-1 concentration was elevated in the presence of severe adhesions. IL-6 levels were appreciably correlated with the grade of endometriosis (P < 0.05), but no significant correlations of either TNF-alpha or IL-1 concentrations were noted with the various grades of endometriosis. Although the precise role of TNF-alpha and IL-1 in adhesion formation is still unclear the results of this study signify that their concentration in the peritoneal fluid is associated with the degree of adhesions present [63].

A study correlating concentrations of mediators in serial samples of peritoneal fluid collected at diagnostic laparoscopy in one group, and at laparoscopy during the first 48 hours after laparoscopic adhesiolysis in a second group, found that the MMP-9 concentration was lower in the follicular phase than the luteal phase of the menstrual cycle. MMP-9 concentration was significantly less in women with pelvic adhesions than in women with a normal pelvis. The MMP-9/TIMP-1 ratio was significantly higher in women with considerable adhesions at second-look laparoscopy compared to women with minimal or no adhesions. The components of extracellular matrix remodeling may play an important part in the adhesion formation/reformation process [64].

Bloody peritoneal fluid (PF) is frequently present in the culde-sac of endometriosis patients and contains an array of biologically active factors. Iwabe T, et al2005 [65], recorded that the concentrations of tumor necrosis factor alpha (TNF-alpha) and interleukin-6 (IL-6) in PF from patients with endometriosis were considerably more elevated than that of patients with endometriosis. There were appreciably positive correlations between the levels of TNF-alpha and IL-6, which also correlated with the number and extent of red color peritoneal endometriosis. TNF-alpha enhanced the expression of IL-6 messenger RNA and protein in endometriotic stromal cells derived from chocolate cyst in a dose-dependent manner [66].

The involvement of T cells in the pathogenesis of endometriosis is a contentious matter. With the aim of investigating the role of T-cell implication in the pathogenesis of endometriosis. Szyllo K et al 2003 [67], conducted a study enrolling women aged 24-46 years with established diagnosis of endometriosis.All the patients studied underwent diagnostic laparoscopy.The distribution of T-lymphocyte subpopulations in peripheral blood (PB), peritoneal fluid (PF) and in endometriotic tissues (ET),as well as cytokines [interleukin (IL)-2, IL-4, IL-10, IL-12, interferon(IFN)-gamma] production by peripheral blood lymphocytes. IFN-gamma, tumor necrosis factor (TNF)-alpha, IL-4 and IL-6 was investigated..The experiments were done before and after 6months treatment with the GnRH-Analogous Goserelin..

Comparison of the lymphocyte subset re-distribution with regard to the American Fertility Society (AFS) stages and scores, showed no differences.. The significant increase in CD4:CD8 ratio, the decrease in the numberof natural killer (NK) cells in PB and the decrease in CD4:CD8 ratio in PF and ETof women with endometriosis was noted. The diminished IFN-gamma secretion by phytohemagglutinim (PHA)-stimulated lymphocytes in vitro derived from women with endometriosis and increased IL-4 production may be the cause of defective immunosurveillance against overgrowth of endometriotic tissues. The diminished NKcells number in PB of women with endometriosis supports such a hypothesis. The increased deposits of proinflammatory IL-6 and TNF-alpha in the T lymphocytes of women with endometriosis may be linked to T-regulatory lymphocyte function and their inability to suppress cell proliferation in endometriosis. GnRH-Analogous Goserelin treatment normalises cytokine production and improves patient recovery. The important functional and phenotypic differences between the lymphocytes from healthy women and women with endometriosis were noted. The diminished IFN-gamma production in relation to reduced NK cells number and the enhanced IL-4 production prior to the treatment and normalisation after the treatment signifies the involvement of the deregulated T-cell system in the growth stimulation and recruitment of endometriotic cells. The increased CD4:CD8 ratio, IL-6, TNF-alpha deposits and diminished anti-inflammatory IL-10 production by lymphocytes may have a role in the pathogenesis of endometriosis, and may secondarily impact the monocyte/macrophage function [67].

Genetic Aspect of Endometriosis:

There is mounting evidence in favour of a genetic basis for endometriosis. Endometriosis is most likely a complex trait, signifying that the disease is the outcome of an interaction between multiple genes and environment. As this condition does not have an obvious Mendelian pattern of inheritance and multiple gene loci confer vulnerability to the condition and interact with each other and the environment [68].

In a study [69] to illustrate the incidence of endometriosis in monozygotic twins. Twins were enrolled via the American Endometriosis Association and the National Endometriosis Society of Great Britain and via British gynecologists. Fourteen twin pairs were concordant for endometriosis, and two were discordant. Nine pairs of twins had moderate-severe endometriosis. These findings add to the mounting body of evidence that suggests endometriosis has a genetic basis [69].

It is well recognized that endometriosis is a condition exhibiting heritable proclivities. Polygenic/multifactorial etiology appears more plausible than Mendelian inheritance. It has also been hypothesized that endometriosis is analogous to neoplasia thus implying it as a multistep phenomenon of clonal origin [70].

Family and twin studies have shown that heritability accounts for endometriosis development to an extent similar to other complex genetic diseases [71].

It is well recognized that daughters or sisters of patients with endometriosis are at higher risk of developing endometriosis themselves; for example, low progesterone levels may be genetic, and may contribute to a hormone imbalance. There is an about 10-fold increased incidence in women with an affected first-degree relative [72]. One study found that in female siblings of patients with endometriosis the relative risk of endometriosis is 5.7:1 versus a control population [73].

With a view to detect molecular differences in the endometrium of women with endometriosis in exploring the pathogenesis and for developing novel approaches for the treatment of the condition. Richard O. Burney et al 2007 [74], conducted global gene expression analysis of endometrium from women with and without moderate/severe stage endometriosis and compared the gene expression signatures in different phases of the menstrual cycle. The study comprised; a) the transcriptome analysis; b) Paralleled gene expression analysis of endometrial specimens; c) gene expression involved in DNA synthesis and cellular mitosis in endometriosis and D) Comparative gene expression analysis of progesterone-regulated genes. The study revealed molecular dysregulation of the proliferative-to-secretory shift in endometrium of women with endometriosis, improved cellular survival and continual expression of genes concerned with DNA synthesis and cellular mitosis at the site of endometriosis. Comparative gene expression analysis of progesterone-regulated genes in secretory phase endometrium established the observation of attenuated progesterone response. Moreover it identified remarkable candidate susceptibility genes that may be linked with endometriosis, including FOXO1A, MIG6, and CYP26A1. Collectively these findings provide a framework for further investigations on causality and mechanisms underlying attenuated progesterone response in endometrium of women with endometriosis [74].

In this context it is pertinent to refer to MicroRNAs (miRNAs), small noncoding RNAs that regulate gene expression, have essential roles in biological processes, including cell differentiation and proliferation. They mostly function as gene silencers and direct either target messenger RNA (mRNA) degradation or translational suppression

It is well known that endometrial cells and glands of the uterus go through cyclic changes under the control of the sex steroid hormones estradiol-17beta and progesterone .Expression of miRNAs in human endometrium has been established,and hence the need to explore the role of miRNAs in modulating the expression of hormonally induced genes prompted the study by Satu Kuokkanen et al 2010 [75] . They found simultaneous differential miRNA and mRNA expression profiles of endometrial cells in the late proliferative and midsecretory phases. It was observed that; 1)differentially expressed mRNAs exposed cell cycle regulation as the most notably enriched pathway in the late proliferative-phase endometrial epithelium ($P = 5.7 \times 10^{-15}$), and 2) the enhancement of WNT signaling pathway in the proliferative phase. There was expression of 12 miRNAs (*MIR29B, MIR29C, MIR30B, MIR30D, MIR31, MIR193A-3P, MIR203, MIR204, MIR200C, MIR210, MIR582-5P,* and *MIR345*) which were appreciably up-regulated in the midsecretory-phase and were predicted to target many cell cycle genes. The suppressor effect of miRNAs on their target mRNA expression was evident from the observed decrease of cyclins and cyclin-dependent kinases, and *E2F3* (a known target of *MIR210*). Thus, their data imply that miRNAs down-regulate the expression of some cell cycle genes in the secretory-phase endometrial epithelium, thus suppressing cell proliferation [75].

Endometriosis is associated with abnormal growth or turn-over of cells, however, the genetic changes involved still awaits further exploration. A study [76], reported that the occurrence of somatic chromosomal changes in severe/late stage endometriosis was studied in four cases of endometriosis .With the aid of alpha-satellite sequence-specific DNA probes for chromosomes 7, 8, 11, 12, 16, 17, and 18, simultaneous two- and three-color FISH were performed to estimate the frequency of monosomic, disomic, and trisomic cells in normal control and endometriotic tissue specimens. One of the endometriosis samples showed , an appreciably higher frequency of monosomy for chromosome 17 (14.8%, $\chi^2_4 = 53.3$, $P < 0.0001$) and 16 (8.8%, $\chi^2_4 = 11.4$, $P < 0.05$). In a second case there was an augmented proportion of cells with chromosome 11 trisomy (14.8%, $\chi^2_4 = 96.2$, $P < 0.0001$) In the third case, a distinct colony of nuclei with chromosome 16 monosomy (14.1%, $\chi^2_4 = 21.39$, $P < 0.005$). A study found Acquired chromosome-specific aneuploidy may be implicated in endometriosis, reflecting clonal expansion of chromosomally abnormal cells. That candidate tumor suppressor genes and oncogenes which have been mapped to chromosomes 11, 16, and 17 imply that deletion or gain of chromosomes has a part to play in the pathogenesis and/or progression of endometriosis [76].

Another study [77], reported a relation between endometriosis and chromosome 10q26, while another study [78], discovered an association with the 7p15.2 region. Admittedly numerous challenges pose problems to genetic investigations on endometriosis because of the diverse manifestations and various forms of endometriosis. The problem is further compounded by factors such as strong gene-environmental interactions that might interfere with approaches to identify genetic variants involved [79].

Both linkage analysis and association studies have been conducted to recognize genetic determinants for the disease. Results from the linkage scan of 1,176 families collected jointly between an Australian and a UK group highlighted an important linkage to a novel susceptibility locus on chromosome 10q26. Gene variants with impact on the disease predilection have been assumed to exist and several candidates have been proposed, but their effects are yet to be established. The major categories of candidate genes studied have been those concerned with detoxification processes, sex steroid biosynthesis and action, immune system regulation. Admittedly numerous challenges pose problems to genetic investigations on endometriosis because of the diverse manifestations and various forms of   endometriosis. Genome-wide association studies that survey most of the genome for causal genetic variants provide the potential for future progress [79].

Recent molecular cytogenetic investigations on endometriotic tissue and endometriosis-derived cell line revealed new proof that acquired chromosome-specific changes may be related to endometriosis, perhaps implying clonal expansion of chromosomally abnormal cells. Molecular DNA studies on the role of loss of heterozygosity in endometriotic lesions has detected candidate tumour suppressor gene loci, including 5q, 6q, 9p, 11q and 22q, that may paticipate in the genesis of endometrioid ovarian cancers.from endometriotic implants . Mutations in the tumour suppressor *PTEN* gene in the endometrioid subtype of epithelial ovarian cancer further indicates that somatic genetic alterations reflect early modification changes in the benign endometriotic cells. It is possible that genetic factors impact individual proneness to endometriosis. There is sign of proof that heritable allelic differences in drug-metabolizing enzymes may have significant part in the pathogenesis of endometriosis [80].

An array of disorders, such as insulin-dependent diabetes mellitus (IDDM), systemic lupus erythematosus (SLE), and pre-eclampsia, , mucous membrane pemphigoid are linked to particular HLA types [81-82], which are regarded as an immune response-related genes.

In view of the lack of any proven connection between endometriosis and HLA antigens and failure of previous studies employing serological analysis to report a statistically significant link between endometriosis and HLA allotype frequency. Keisuke Ishii et al 2002 [83], investigated to detect the possible relation between endometriosis HLA allotype frequency. In their study noted that the prevalence of the HLA-

DRB1*1403 allele was significantly greater in patients with endometriosis than in the general controls. They [83] observed that the prevalence of HLA-DQB1*0301 in the former group was 16.3% relative to 8.3% in the overall control group and 7.7% in the females of the control group. The frequency of the HLA-DQB1*0301 allele was appreciably greater in endometriosis patients compared with the general controls Association in the frequencies of DPB1 alleles between the patients and controls was hardly noticeable. Thus their study lends support to imply that HLA systems may be implicated in the aetiology of endometriosis [83].

Oxford Endometriosis Gene Study (OXEGENE) is designed to discover whether there is a genetic cause for endometriosis, and to identify susceptibility loci involved in the development of endometriosis using the linkage analysis. DNA from sisters with surgically confirmed r-AFS stage II-IV disease and their parents are being collected to perform a genome-wide screen. There were 571 Families, 886 patients and 65 collaborators involving this study until the time that this manuscript was in preparation.

Endometriosis is an intricate disorder that has long been recognized as presenting heritable tendencies, with recurrence risks of 5-7% for first-degree relatives. Familial and epidemiologic studies substantiate its genetic basis and the disorder is of polygenic/multifactorial inheritance.

The current investigational challenge is to determine the number and location of causative genes. Recent advances in molecular technology make identification and elucidation of these genes now possible [84].

Two genetic associations with endometriosis have been reported: 1) Polymorphism in galactose-1-phosphate uridyl transferase (GALT); 2) Null mutation in Glutathione S-transferase M1 (GSTM1) [85-86]. Enzymes belonging to the glutathione S-transferase family are involved in the two stage of detoxification of 2,3,7,8-Tetraachlorodibenzo-p-Dioxin (Dioxin) which is a potential pollutant for endometriosis development [85-86].

It will be of much interest to refer to the controversies surrounding the glutathione S-transferases (GST) M1/T1–endometriosis association. In view of the debate a meta-analysis of the GSTM1/GSTT1 genetic association studies of endometriosis was performed [87]. This meta-analysis involved 14 GSTM1 studies with 1539 cases and 1805 controls and nine GSTT1 studies with 746 cases and 834 controls, respectively,and it showed considerable heterogeneities among studies. There was no evidence that women with GSTM1 null genotype have augmented risk of developing endometriosis as compared with women with other genotypes. For GSTT1, the risk associated with the null genotype is 29% higher than other genotypes. Nevertheless, the author has cautioned that even this approximation should be viewed with skepticism as regards its questionable statistical significance [87].

To explore a possible connection between endometriosis, Müllerian anomalies, and possession of the N314D allele of the gene for galactose-1-phosphate uridyl transferase (GALT), a study was conducted and it comprised 33 women with endometriosis The patients were DNA tested for the N314D mutation of GALT. Compared with endometriosis cases without the N314D allele, those cases with the allele tended to have more advanced disease and a family history of endometriosis. This in fact throws some light on one of the causes of endometriosis, in turn due to Muelleriam obstruction. Thus they were led them to infer that endometriosis may arise due to defects of canalization of the cervix leading to cervical stenosis and retrograde menstruation. The relevance of the N314D mutation, via this model, may derive from an association between abnormalities of galactose metabolism and vaginal agenesis which represents a canalization defect of the vaginal plate of the Müllerian tubercle, the same structure which gives rise to the cervix [88].

An investigation by Mayumi Morizane et al 2004 [89] was performed to look at the frequency of glutathione S-transferase M1 and T1 (GSTM1 and GSTT1) null mutations in women with endometriosis in a Japanese population. The study enrolled one hundred fourteen unrelated women with endometriosis Samples of Umbilical cord blood samples from 179 female newborn infants served as population controls. Genomic DNA isolated from endometriosis patients and controls were subjected to multiple polymerase chain reactions to determine the

GSTM1 and GSTT1 genotypes. There were no significant differences in the frequencies of the GSTM1 (P = .83, odds ratio 0.95) and GSTT1 (P = .24, odds ratio 0.75) null mutations between endometriosis patients and controls. Their findings do not support that the GSTM1 and GSTT1 null mutations are likely to be associated with an increased risk of endometriosis in a Japanese population [89].

Endometriosis is well established as a condition showing heritable tendencies. Polygenic/multifactorial etiology appears far more likely to be the etiology than Mendelian inheritance. The current task is to determine the number and location of genes responsible for endometriosis. The revision should include the basis for concluding that endometriosis is a genetic disorder of polygenic/multifactorial inheritance and outline selected strategies for identifying the number and location of causative genes. It also exemplifies their approach to testing the hypothesis that endometriosis bears similarity to neoplasia and, thus, is a multistep phenomenon of clonal origin [70].

A few words of proteomics and its usefulness in the study endometriosis with new proteins that have a potential role in the initiation and progression of endometriosis: it also serves as stage or for more investigations on mechanisms implicated in the pathogenesis of endometriosis.

The detection of molecular differences in the endometrium of women with endometriosis is an essential in the right direction of exploring the pathogenesis of this condition and for developing new strategies for the treatment of the condition. Rai P, et al 2010 [90] studied protein expression analysis of eutopic endometrium from women with and without endometriosis it was observed that . it revealed molecular dysregulation of more than 70 proteins in the proliferative phase of eutopic endometrium in stage IV and secretory phase of stage II, III and IV endometriosis Mass spectrometry detected , 48 proteins spots which were consistently differentially expressed from stage II to IV endometriosis were identified. The differentially expressed proteins include structural proteins, proteins involved in stress response, protein-folding and protein-turnover, immunity, energy production, signal transduction, RNA biogenesis, protein biosynthesis, and nuclear proteins. Immunoblot and immunohistochemical analyses confirmed the observed changes in eight representative proteins. The present study provides identification of new players that have a potential role in the initiation and progression of endometriosis and also sets a framework for further investigations on mechanisms underlying the pathogenesis of endometriosis [90].

Familial clustering in Rhesus monkeys

Familial tendency of disease supporting the hypothesis that endometriosis has a genetic basis was discovered in these studies. The clinical features at surgery and histological characteristics of the disease in the rhesus monkey resemble those in human. Therefore, the clearer understanding of the epidemiology and inheritability of the disease may emerge from studying spontaneous endometriosis in rhesus monkey colonies (Macaca Mulatta). Oxford Group is collaborating with California Regional Primate Research Center (CRPRC) and Wisconsin Regional Primate Research Center (WRPRC) to study the epidemiology and inheritability of endometriosis. They have identified 121 (8.3%) affected rhesus monkeys among the autopsy records of the 1459 female animals that they died, aged 4 years of more, in the colony between 1982-1996 at CRPRC. They are trying to determine the familial tendency in these affected animals by analyzing the entire colony records over 9000 females from 1965-1977. Hadfield et al studied the autopsy records of 399 rhesus monkeys that died in the WRPRC colony between 1980 and 1995 and reported a prevalence rate of 20% in animals aged 4 years or older at death and 29% in animals aged 10 years or older at death [91].

The development of an animal model of endometriosis is vital for the study of disease pathogenesis and therapeutic intercession. These models will improve the methods of evaluation the causes for the subfertility associated with disease and offer the most important justification of treatment modulators. Presently rodents and non-human primate models have been developed, but each model has its own constraints They have summarized the recent findings and theories on the pathogenesis of endometriosis ,disease progression and the efficacy of therapeutic targets using the experimental induced model of endometriosis in the baboon (*Papio anubis*) [91]..

The chicken chorioallantoic membrane (CAM) model can be regarded as an animal model in the broader sense. Although innovatively , it had been developed to study the invasive, metastatic and angiogenic potential of neoplastic cells [92]. It is now an established as a model for endometriosis by culturing fragments of human endometrial tissue on the basal layer of the CAM of fertilized chicken eggs after prior incubation for 7–10 days [93-94]. Endometrial fragments from the proliferative and secretory phase of the menstrual cycle as well as the menstrual endometrium invade across the epithelium into the mesenchymal layer and develop endometriosis-like lesions in this layer of the CAM within 3 days after grafting of the human tissue. It was shown that these endometrial fragments needed to contain intact glandular structures as well as stromal components [92-94].

Stem cell theory of endometriosis:

Adult stem cells are thought to be responsible for the high regenerative capacity of the human endometrium, and have been implicated in the pathology of endometriosis and endometrial carcinoma.

The RNA-binding protein Musashi-1 is associated with maintenance and asymmetric cell division of neural and epithelial progenitor cells. Götte, M.et al 2008 [95], investigated expression and localization of Musashi-1 in endometrial, endometrio tic and endometrial carcinoma tissue specimens of 46 patients. qPCR revealed significantly increased *Musashi-1* mRNA expression in the endometrium compared to the myometrium. Musashi-1 protein expression presented as nuclear or cytoplasmic immunohistochemical staining of single cells in endometrial glands, and of single cells and cell groups in the endometrial stroma. Immunofluorescence microscopy revealed colocalization of Musashi-1 with its molecular target Notch-1 and telomerase. In proliferative endometrium, the proportion of Musashi-1-positive cells in the basalis layer was significantly increased 1.5 fold in the stroma, and three-fold in endometrial glands compared to the functionalis. The number of Musashi-1 expressing cell groups was significantly increased (four-fold) in proliferative compared to secretory endometrium. Musashi-1 expressing stromal cell and cell group numbers were significantly increased (five-fold) in both endometriotic and endometrial carcinoma tissue compared to secretory endometrium. A weak to moderate, diffuse cytoplasmic glandular staining was seen in 50% of the endometriosis cases and in 75% of the endometrioid carcinomas compared to complete absence in normal endometrial samples. Their findings highlight the importance the role of Musashi-1-expressing endometrial progenitor cells in proliferating endometrium, endometriosis and endometrioid uterine carcinoma, and uphold the perception of a stem cell origin of endometriosis and endometrial carcinoma [95].

A retrospective analysis on necropsy records from a rhesus monkey colony of 66 monkeys with histologically verified endometriosis and 248 control subjects. to assess the age-related incidence of endometriosis revealed that the incidence of endometriosis increases progressively across the life span, eventually affecting 21-45% of aged monkeys over 20 years of age [96].

While it is common to see endometriosis in humans it has also been observed in animals. This is evident from studies that follow. An observational longitudinal study was conducted by D'Hooghe TM, et al [97], at the Institute of Primate Research, Nairobi (Kenya), using 24 baboons with laparoscopically confirmed normal pelves underwent 67 serial laparoscopies for a variable length of follow-up,from one month to 32 months. Considering the variable length of follow-up, they used life-table analysis to calculate the cumulative incidence of endometriosis. The cumulative incidence of minimal endometriosis (proven by histology) was 64% up to 32 months of follow-up. The eight baboons that developed confirmed endometriosis were followed over longer periods of time and had undergone more laparoscopies than the animals that did not develop the condition.Their studies concluded that there is a high incidence of minimal endometriosis in baboons, which increases with the duration of follow-up and the number of repeat laparoscopies [97].

Sherry E. Rier et al 1993 [98], determined the incidence of endometriosis in a colony of rhesus monkeys constantly exposed to 2,3,7,8-tetrachlorodibenzo-p-dioxin (TCDD or dioxin) for 4 years. Ten years after cessation of dioxin treatment, endometriosis was diagnosed at laparoscopy and the severity of disease was assessed. The incidence of endometriosis was directly correlated with dioxin exposure and the severity of disease was dependent upon the dose administered ($p <$ 0.001). Three of 7 animals exposed to 5 ppt dioxin (43%) and 5 of 7 animals exposed to 25 ppt dioxin (71%) had moderate to severe endometriosis. In contrast, the frequency of disease in the control group was 33%, similar to an overall prevalence of 30% in 304 rhesus monkeys with no dioxin exposure. This 15-year study implies that latent female reproductive abnormalities may be associated with dioxin exposure in the rhesus [98].

Environmental factors

Our body works it's best to cope with hundreds of synthetic chemicals everyday, if any thing goes wrong during this process, free radicals form as well as increasing the risk of some of the cells of the peritoneum to develop into endometrial cells.

Studies have provided important information about environmental factors and their potential influence on development of endometriosis [99]. For example, rhesus monkeys exposed to whole-body proton irradiation have a higher frequency of endometriosis than controls (53% vs 26%) [100]. Also, rhesus monkeys exposed to 5–25 ppm dioxin per day for 4 years developed endometriosis that was dose-dependent in staging [99-101].

Extrapolation to women was initially thought to be epidemiologically plausible, especially with the publication of a report that Belgium, with the highest dioxin pollution in the world, has the highest incidence of endometriosis as well as the highest prevalence of severe endometriosis [102]. However, two subsequent prospective studies from Italy and Belgium found no significantly increased risk of endometriosis in women who have been exposed to dioxin [99, 103-104].

To date, there has been no epidemiological study definitively linking one class of chemicals to the risk of endometriosis, although oestrogen-like compounds in the environment have been suggested [105]. The lack of a definitive link is not surprising because people are exposed to a multiplicity of chemicals, with mechanisms of action that might vary with dose, timing of exposure (in utero, childhood, peripubertally, adult), route of exposure, and synergy with other chemicals, [105] all proceeding against unique genetic backgrounds [99].

A survey by the Centers For Disease Control and Prevention (National Report on Human Exposure to Environmental Chemicals) is now under way; biomonitoring of 145 chemicals in 2500 people in the USA is carried out every 2 years [99]. A major challenge is to relate the data to disease risk. Although biomonitoring for specific chemicals could be interesting, the effect on health, including the development of endometriosis, will probably take years to elucidate, if there is indeed causality. Recent reviews underscore the roles of the toxic chemicals, lifestyle, and reproductive health; [99, 106-107].

Few studies that have been undertaken suggest that lifestyle and dietary factors may be associated with susceptibility to developing endometriosis [108-110] The results of these epidemiological studies found that a diet high in fruit and vegetables and low in meat products was protective against developing endometriosis. Additionally, women with few or no children and low body mass index (BMI) were at a higher risk of developing endometriosis.

Other authors have suggested that exposure to synthetic compounds such as dioxin and other polychlorinated biphenyls (PCBs) could lead to the development of endometriosis due to their effects as endocrine

disruptors [112-113] Dioxin is a by product of the chlorine bleaching

process used in the wood pulp processing industry, this also includes the

manufacture of tampons which is thought to be a major source of dioxin

exposure in women. However, the associations with dioxin are mainly

based on animal data [114-116] which some authors criticise for poor

study design and data analysis [117] Human data on dioxin exposure

and endometriosis risk is scant and in some cases appear contradictory.

For example, a study reported that the incidence of deeply infiltrating

endometriosis in Belgium, reportedly the highest in the world, correlates

with high dioxin exposure through breast milk [118]. However, another

study assessed massive dioxin exposure from the Seveso incident in Italy

during the summer of 1976, whereby a chemical manufacturing plant

accidentally released 1Kg of dioxin into the atmosphere, showering the

neighbouring residential areas with dioxin. Although extremely high

levels of dioxin contamination were found in soil and water samples, no

significant increase in endometriosis incidence were observed, even after

a 26 year follow up study [119] Despite reported increased serum dioxin

levels [120-121] and increased serum levels of bisphenols [121]

observed in endometriosis patients, a conclusive association between

environmental toxicant exposure and increased risk of developing

endometriosis has yet to be established. Given the variety and conflicting

notions pertaining to the origin and development of endometriosis, it becomes clear why endometriosis is often referred to as the *'disease of theories'* [122].

Xenoestrogen overload: Xenoestrogens are but environmental chemicals with estrogenic activity [123]. Xenohormones are new, and have only been known in since about 1991. They are by-products of manufacturing processes, such as synthetic chemicals, which simulate the effect of natural estrogen produced by our body.
Some of these Xenoestrogens like DDE (a metabolite of DDT) may persist in the body fat for decades. Many of these mimicking hormones which were once thought to occur in pesticides were regarded as inert materials. Xenoestrogens,have attracted considerable attention theoretically agreement is centred around the fact that such compounds, in high doses, may induce developmental, reproductive and tumorigenic effects together with a critical appraisal of methods to detect and quantitate the estrogenic activity of synthetic and naturally occurring chemicals [123].

The manner in which Xenoestrogens are implicated in the etiology of endometriosis.is briefly described below. During the rush of estrogen at the commencement of menstrual cycle, over-production of xenoestrogen induces hormone imbalance leading to over-stimulation of certain hormones, inducing metaplasia of peritoneal lining cells into endometrial cells.

Overdose of Environmental toxins from food air, or contact through skin cause hormonal imbalance leading to xenoestrogens enhancing the risk of endometriosis. In addition Xenoestrogens being toxic tend to weaken the immune system Overdose of xenoestrogens not only disturbs the production of natural estrogen from our body, but it also predisposes to the generation of free radicals and weakens the immune system to defend against any bacteria and virus as well as implanting endometrial cells in unusual sites in the body. Again overload of xenoestrogen through food consumption may stimulate high level of estrogen production leading to hormone imbalance as well as augmenting the risk of endometriosis., According to the coelomic metaplasia theory Xenoestrogens toxify and disrupt the normal cell development favouring the risk of some of the peritoneal cells to develop into endometrial cells. Finally Xenoestrogens by augmenting the production of estrogen induce hormone imbalance resulting in disruption of menstrual cycle promoting the development of growth of endometriosis. Endometriosis as is well known is an estrogen-dependent disease, c-fos is an early transcription factor that has been documented to be linked to estradiol-dependent cell proliferation. Morsch DM, et al 2009 [124], performed a study to assess the c-fos gene and protein expression in pelvic endometriotic implants in comparison to normal endometrium from infertile women. This open, prospective and controlled study comprising 15 infertile women with endometriosis and

19 control infertile women. Endometrial and endometriotic biopsies were performed at the follicular phase and the samples were processed for RT-PCR and immunohistochemistry.). c-fos gene expression was more elevated in endometriotic implants (1.32 +/- 0.13; P = 0.011) than in eutopic endometrium from patients with endometriosis (0.97 +/- 0.11) or from the control group (0.91 +/- 0.05). Besides, immunohistochemistry revealed a more copious distribution of c-Fos in the stroma of endometriotic tissue relative to eutopic endometrium. These findings imply the role of c-fos may in the molecular mechanisms of estrogen action on the initiation and evolution of endometriosis [124].

Xenoestrogen bisphenol A (BPA) simulates estrogen both in vivo and in vitro. One of the explicit objectives of the study by R Steinmetz, et al 1998 [125], was to characterize the short term effects of BPA on cell proliferation and c-fos expression in the uterus and vagina, Treatment with single high doses of BPA induced cell proliferation in the uterus and vagina of ovariectomized F344 rats. By quantitative RT-PCR it was shown that both BPA and E2 increased c-fos messenger RNA levels in the uterus 14- to 16-fold within 2 h, which returned to basal levels after 6 h [125]. It is relevant at this juncture to refer to the studies of Morsch DM, et al 2009 [124] which imply the role of c-fos may in the molecular mechanisms of estrogen action on the initiation and evolution of endometriosis.

The immune system which is under composite control can react promptly to the environment., Recent findings emphasize the likely implication of environmental xenobiotic chemicals which can alter normal immune function. Currently much attention is focused on chemicals which influence sex steroids in the genesis of immune diseases; this stems from the increased occurrence of autoimmune disease in women, the gender variation in the immune response, as well as the immunomodulatory influence of sex steroids, Furthermore, recent reports indicate that certain environmental chemicals can exert their influence on nuclear hormone receptors, besides sex hormone receptors, and affectt immune reactions [126].

References

1. <u>Seli E,Berkkanoglu Arici A</u>M. Pathogenesis of endometriosis. <u>Obstetrics and Gynecology Clinics of North America</u> 2003; 30(1):41-61.

2. Oral, E. & Arici, A.. Pathogenesis of endometriosis. Obstetric and Gynecology Clinics 1997; 24 (2): 219-233.

3. Matsuura, K., Ohtake, H., Katabuchi, H. & Okamura, H. Coelomic Metaplasia Theory of Endometriosis: Evidence from in Vivo Studies and an in vitro experimental Model. Gynecologic and Obstetric Investigation 1999; 47 (Suppl1): 18-22.

4. Sampson JA. Ovarian hematomas of endometrial type (perforating hemorrhagic cysts of the ovary) and implantation adenomas of endometrial type. Boston Med Surg J 1922; 186: 445–73.

5. Sampson JA. Peritoneal endometriosis due to menstrual dissemination of endometrial tissue into the peritoneal cavity. Am J Obst Gynecol 1927; 14: 442–69.

6. Vinatier, D., Cosson, M. & Dufour, P. Is endometriosis an endometrial disease? European Journal of Obstetrics, Gynaecology and Reproductive Biology 2000; 91(2): 113-25.

7. Keetle, WC. & Stein, RJ. The viability of the cast off menstrual endometrium. American Journal of Obstetrics and Gynecology 1951; 61: 440.

8. Kale, S., Shuster, M. & Sahmgold, I. Endometrioma in a caesarean scar: case report and review of literature. American Journal of Obstetrics and Gynecology 1971; 111: 596.

9. Scott RB, Te Linde RW, Wharton LR Jr. Further studies on experimental endometriosis. Am J Obstet Gynecol. 1953; 66:1082.

10. Liu DT, Hitchcock A. Endometriosis: its association with retrograde menstruation, dysmenorrhoea and tubal pathology. Br J Obstet Gynaecol. Aug 1986; 93(8):859-62.

11.Kruitwagen RF, Poels LG, Willemsen WN, de Ronde IJ, Jap PH, Rolland R. Endometrial epithelial cells in peritoneal fluid during the early follicular phase. Fertil Steril. Feb 1991; 55(2):297-303.

12. D'Hooghe TM, Bambra CS, Raeymaekers BM, Koninckx PR. Increased prevalence and recurrence of retrograde menstruation in baboons with spontaneous endometriosis. Hum Reprod. Sep 1996; 11(9):2022-5.

13. Thomas M. D'Hooghe, Charanjit S, Barbara M. Raeymaekers, Inge De Jonge, Jo M. Lauweryns and P. R. Koninckx. Intrapelvic injection of menstrual endometrium causes endometriosis in baboons (Papio cynocephalus and Papio Anubis). American Journal of Obstetrics and Gynecology 1995; 173(1): 125-134.

14. Wu MY, Ho HN.The role of cytokines in endometriosis. Am J Reprod Immunol 2003; 49(5):285-96.

15. Osamu Yoshino, Yutaka Osuga, Kaori Koga, Yasushi Hirota, Tetsuya Hirata, Xie Ruimeng, Li Na, Tetsu Yano, Osamu Tsutsum, Yuji Taketani. FR 167653, a p38 mitogen-activated protein kinase inhibitor, suppresses the development of endometriosis in a murine model. Journal of Reproductive Immunology 2006; 72(1-2): 85-93.

16. Philippe R. Koninckz, Anastasia Ussia. Epidemiology of endometriosis. Book chapter written April 2003; 5: 1-16.

17. Redwine D. Was Sampson wrong? Fertil.Steril. 2002;78:686.

18. Koninckx PR, Barlow D, Kennedy S. Implantation versus infiltration:

the Sampson versus the endometriotic disease theory. Gynecol. Obstet.Invest 1999;47 Suppl 1:3-9.

19. Halme J, Hammond MG, Hulka JF, Raj SG, Talbert LM. Retrograde menstruation in healthy women and in patients with endometriosis. Obstet Gynecol 1984; 64:151-154.

20. Kitawaki J, Kado N, Ishihara H, Koshiba H, Kitaoka Y, Honjo H. Endometriosis: the pathophysiology as an estrogen-dependent disease. J Steroid Biochem Mol Biol. 2002; 83(1-5):149-55.

21. Serdar E. Bulun, Zongjuan Fang, Gonca Imir, Bilgin Gurates, Mitsutoshi Tamura, Bertan Yilmaz, David Langoi, Sanober Amin, Sijun Yang and Santanu Deb. Aromatase in endometriosis Semin Reprod Med. 2004; 22(1):

22. Noble LS, Simpson ER, Johns A, Bulun SE. Aromatase expression in endometriosis. J Clin Endocrinol Metab 1996; 81:174-179

23. Bulun SE, Simpson ER, Word RA. Expression of the CYP19 gene and its product aromatase cytochrome P450 in human leiomyoma tissues and cells in culture. J Clin Endocrinol Metab 1994; 78:736-743

24. Noble LS, Takayama K, Zeitoun KM, et al. Prostaglandin E_2 stimulates aromatase expression in endometriosis-derived stromal cells. J Clin Endocrinol Metab 1997; 82:600-606.

25. Michael MD, Michael LF, Simpson ER. A CRE-like sequence that binds CREB and contributes to cAMP-dependent regulation of the proximal promoter of the human aromatase P450 (CYP19) gene. Mol Cell Endocrinol 1997; 134:147-156.

26. Michael MD, Kilgore MW, Morohashi KI, Simpson ER. Ad4BP/SF-1 regulates cyclic AMP-induced transcription from the proximal promoter (PII) of the human aromatase P450 (CYP19) gene in the ovary. J Biol Chem 1995; 270:13561-13566.

27. Ackerman GE, Smith ME, Mendelson CR, MacDonald PC, Simpson ER. Aromatization of androstenedione by human adipose tissue stromal cells in monolayer culture. J Clin Endocrinol Metab 1981;53:412-417

28. MacDonald PC, Rombaut RP, Siiteri PK. Plasma precursors of estrogen, I: Extent of conversion of plasma Δ^4-androstenedione to estrone in normal males and non-pregnant normal, castrate and adrenalectomized females. J Clin Endocrinol Metab 1967;27:1103-1111

29. MacDonald PC, Edman CD, Hemsell DL, Porter JC, Siiteri PK. Effect of obesity on conversion of plasma androstenedione to estrone in postmenopausal women with and without endometrial cancer. Am J Obstet Gynecol 1978;130:448-455

30. Simpson ER, Mahendroo MS, Means GD, et al. Aromatase

cytochrome P450, the enzyme responsible for estrogen biosynthesis. Endocr Rev 1994;15:342-355

31. Noble LS, Simpson ER, Johns A, Bulun SE. Aromatase expression in endometriosis. J Clin Endocrinol Metab 1996; 81:174-179

32. Zeitoun K, Takayama K, Michael MD, Bulun SE. Stimulation of aromatase P450 promoter (II) activity in endometriosis and its inhibition in endometrium are regulated by competitive binding of SF-1 and COUP-TF to the same cis-acting element. Mol Endocrinol 1999;13:239-253

33. Noble LS, Takayama K, Zeitoun KM, et al. Prostaglandin E_2 stimulates aromatase expression in endometriosis-derived stromal cells. J Clin Endocrinol Metab 1997;82:600-606

34.Tamura M, Deb S, Sebastian S, Okamura K, Bulun SE. Estrogen up-regulates cyclooxygenase-2 via estrogen receptor in human uterine microvascular endothelial cells. Fertil Steril 2004. In press.

35. Khorram O, Taylor RN, Ryan IP, Schall TJ, Landers DV. Peritoneal fluid concentrations of the cytokine RANTES correlate with the severity of endometriosis. Am J Obstet Gynecol 1993;169:1545-1549

36. Sharpe-Timms KL, Penney LL, Zimmer RL, Wright JA, Zhang Y, Surewicz K. Partial purification and amino acid sequence analysis of

endometriosis protein-II (ENDO-II) reveals homology with tissue inhibitor of metalloproteinases-1 (TIMP-1). J Clin Endocrinol Metab 1995;80:3784-3787.

37. Hill JA. Immunology and endometriosis. Fertil Steril 1992; 58:262-264

38. Kitawaki J, Kado N, Ishihara H, Koshiba H, Kitaoka Y, Honjo H. Endometriosis: the pathophysiology as an estrogen-dependent disease. J Steroid Biochem Mol Biol. 2002; 83(1-5):149-55.

39. Salem ML. Estrogen, a double-edged sword: modulation of TH1- and TH2-mediated inflammations by differential regulation of TH1/TH2 cytokine production. Curr Drug Targets Inflamm Allergy. 2004 Mar;3(1):97-104.

40. Verena Mönckedieck,Carolin Sannecke,Bettina Husen, Michael Kumbartsk Rainer Kimmig, Martin Tötsch, Elke Winterhagerd Ruth Grümmer. Progestins inhibit expression of MMPs and of angiogenic factors in human ectopic endometrial lesions in a mouse model Mol. Hum. Reprod 2009; 15(10): 633-643.

41. J. Szamatowicz, P. Laudański, and I. Tomaszewska. Matrix metalloproteinase-9 and tissue inhibitor of matrix metalloproteinase-1: a possible role in the pathogenesis of endometriosis Hum. Reprod 2002; 17

(2): 284-288.

42. Seli E. Endometriosis: interaction of immune and endocrine systems. Semin Reprod Med. 2003; 21(2):135-44.

43. Batt RE, Smith RA, Buck Louis GM, Martin DC, Chapron C, Koninckx PR, Yeh J. Müllerianosis. Histol Histopathol. 2007; 22(10):1161-6.

44. Batt RE, Smith RA, Buck GM, Severino MF, Naples JD. Müllerianosis Prog Clin Biol Res 1990; 323:413-26.

45. Schenken RS, Johnson JV, Riehl RM. c-myc protooncogene polypeptide expression in endometriosis. Am J Obstet Gynecol. 1991; 164(4):1031-6;

46. May K, Becker CM. Endometriosis and angiogenesis. Minerva Ginecol. 2008; 60(3):24.

47. Matsuura K, Ohtake H, Katabuchi H, Okamura H. Coelomic metaplasia theory of endometriosis: evidence from in vivo studies and an in vitro experimental model. Gynecol Obstet Invest. 1999; 47 Suppl 1:18-20.

48. I. Velasco ruiz, A. Campos Ferrer, P. Acién Alvarez, F. Quereda seguí. Antiendometrial antibodies and endometriosis. Obestet Gynecol 1990; 75(6):914-8.

49. Mathur S, Garza DE, Smith LF. Endometrial autoantigens eliciting immunoglobulin IgG, IgA, and IgM responses in endometriosis. Fertil Steril. 1990; 54(1):56-63.

50. Pillai S, Zhou GX, Arnaud P, Jiang H, Butler WJ, Zhang H. Antibodies to endometrial transferrin and alpha 2-Heremans Schmidt (HS) glycoprotein in patients with endometriosis. Am J Reprod Immunol 1996; 35(5):483-94.

51. D'Cruz OJ, Wild RA, Haas GG Jr, Reichlin M. Antibodies to carbonic anhydrase in endometriosis: prevalence, specificity, and relationship to clinical and laboratory parameters. Fertil Steril 1996; 66(4):547-56.

52. Sundqvist J., Falconer H., Seddighzadeh M., Vodolazkaia A., Fassbender A., Kyama C., Bokor A., Stephansson O., Padyukov L., Gemzell-Danielsson K., D'Hooghe T.M. Endometriosis and autoimmune disease: association of susceptibility to moderate/severe endometriosis with CCL21 and HLA-DRB1. Fertil. Steril. 2011; 95:437-440.

53. Rasheed K, Atta H, Taha TF, Azmy O, Sabry D, Selim M, El-Sawaf A, Bibars M, Ramzy A, El-Garf W, Anwar JSRM Vol VI Issue: 3.

54. Dmowski WP, Gebel HM, Braun DP. The role of cell-mediated immunity in pathogenesis of endometriosis. Am J Reprod Immunol. 1996; 35(2):118-22.

55. Chi-Chen Chang, Yao-Yuan Hsieh, Fuu-Jen Tsai, Chang-Hai Tsai, Horng-Der Tsai, Cheng-Chieh Lin. The proline form of p53 codon 72 polymorphism is associated with endometriosis. Fertility and Sterility 2002; 77(1): 43-45.

56. Vercellini P, Trecca D, Oldani S, Fracchiolla NS, Neri A, Crosignani PG. Analysis of p53 and ras gene mutations in endometriosis. Gynecol Obstet Invest 1994; 38:70-1.

57. Sakamoto T, Repasky WT, Uchida K, Hirata A, Hirata F. Modulation of cell death pathways to apoptosis and necrosis of H2O2-treated rat thymocytes by lipocortin I. Biochem Biophys Res Commun 1996; 220: 643-647.

58. Chun-yan, LANG Jing-he, LIU Hai-yuan and ZHOU Hui-mei. Expression of Annexin-1 in patients with endometriosis. Chinese Medical Journal 2008; 121(10):927-931.

59. Radke S, Austermann J, Russo-Marie F, Gerke V, Rescher U. Specific association of annexin 1 with plasma membrane-resident and internalized EGF receptors mediated through the protein core domain. FEBS Lett 2004; 578 (1-2): 95-98.

60. Skouteris GG, Schröder CH. The hepatocyte growth factor receptor kinase-mediated phosphorylation of lipocortin-1 transduces the proliferating signal of the hepatocyte growth factor. J Biol Chem 1996;

271: 27266-27273.

61. Varticovski L, Chahwala SB, Whitman M, Cantley L, Schindler D, Chow EP, et al. Location of sites in human lipocortin I that are phosphorylated by protein tyrosine kinases and protein kinases A and C. Biochemistry 1988; 27: 3682-3690.

62. Dmowski WP. Immunological aspects of endometriosis. Int J Gynaecol Obstet 1995; 50 (Suppl 1): S3-S10.

63. Cheong YC, Shelton JB, Laird SM, Richmond M, Kudesia G, Li TC, Ledger WL. IL-1, IL-6 and TNF-alpha concentrations in the peritoneal fluid of women with pelvic adhesions. Hum Reprod. 2002, 17(1): 69-75.

64. Cheong YC, Shelton JB, Laird SM, Li TC, Ledger WL,Cooke ID. Peritoneal fluid concentrations of matrix metalloproteinase-9, tissue inhibitor of metalloproteinase-1, and transforming growth factor-beta in women with pelvic adhesions. Fertil Steril 2003; 79(5): 1168-75.

65. Iwabe T, Harada T, Terakawa N. Role of cytokines in endometriosis-associated infertility. Gynecol Obstet Invest. 2002; 53 Suppl 1:19-25.

66. Hammond MG, Oh ST, Anners J, Surrey ES, Halme J. The effect of growth factors on the proliferation of human endometrial stromal cells in culture. Am J Obstet Gynecol 1993; 168:1131-6.

67. Szyllo K, Tchorzewski H, Banasik M, Glowacka E, Lewkowicz P, Kamer-Bartosinska The involvement of T lymphocytes in the pathogenesis of endometriotic tissues overgrowth in women with endometriosis. Mediators Inflamm. 2003; 12(3):131-8.

68. Erkut Attar,. Current Concepts and Research in the Pathogenesis of Endometriosis. http://www.endometriosiszone.org. Accessed 19th March 2014.

69. Hadfield RM, Mardon HJ, Barlow DH, Kennedy SH. Endometriosis in monozygotic twins.Fertil Steril. 1997 Nov;68(5):941-2.

70. Simpson JL, Bischoff FZ. Heritability and molecular genetic studies of endometriosis. Ann N Y Acad Sci. 2002; 955:239-51.

71. Vigano P, Somigliana E, Vignali M, Busacca M, Blasio AM. Genetics of endometriosis: current status and prospects. Front Biosci. 2007; 12:3247-55.

72. Dharmesh Kapoor and Willy Davila. 'Endometriosis', eMedicine (2005).

73. Kashima K, Ishimaru T, Okamura H, et al. Familial risk among Japanese patients with endometriosis. International Journal of Gynaecology and Obstetrics 2004; 84 (1): 61–4.

74. Richard O. Burney, Said Talbi, Amy E. Hamilton, Kim Chi Vo, Mette Nyegaard, Camran R. Nezhat, Bruce A. Lessey and Linda C. Giudice 2007 Gene Expression Analysis of Endometrium Reveals Progesterone Resistance and Candidate Susceptibility Genes in Women with Endometriosis. Endocrinology 2007; 148(8): 3814-3826.

75.Satu Kuokkanen, Bo Chen, Laureen Ojalvo, Lumie Benard, Nanette Santoro, and Jeffrey W. Pollard. Genomic Profiling of MicroRNAs and Messenger RNAs Reveals Hormonal Regulation in MicroRNA Expression in Human Endometrium1 Biology of Reproduction 2010; 82(4): 791-801.

76. Jong-Chul Shin, Helen L. Ross, Sherman Elias, Dianne D. Nguyen, Dorothy Mitchell-Leef, Joe Leigh Simpson and F. Z. Bischoff. Detection of chromosomal aneuploidy in endometriosis by multi-color fluorescence in situ hybridization (FISH Human Genetics 1997; 100 (3-4): 401-406.

77. Treloar SA, Wicks J, Nyholt DR, et al. Genomewide linkage study in 1,176 affected sister pair families identifies a significant susceptibility locus for endometriosis on chromosome 10q26. American Journal of Human Genetics 2005; 77 (3): 365–76.

78. Painter JN et al. "Genome-wide association study identifies a locus at 7p15.2 associated with endometriosis". Nature Genetics 2010; 43 (1): 51–54.

79. Vigano P, Somigliana E, Vignali M, Busacca M, Blasio AM. Genetics of endometriosis: current status and prospects. Front Biosci. 2007; 12:3247-55.

80. Farideh Z. Bischoff, and Joe Leigh Simpson. Heritability and molecular genetic studies of endometriosis. Hum. Reprod. Update 2000; 6 (1): 37-44.

81. Setterfield, J., Theron, J., Vaughan, R., Welsh, K., Mallon, E., Wojnarowska, F., Challacombe, S. and Black, M. (2001), Mucous membrane pemphigoid: HLA-DQB1*0301 is associated with all clinical sites of involvement and may be linked to antibasement membrane IgG production. British Journal of Dermatology 2001; 145: 406–414.

82. F Pociot, and M F McDermott. Genetics of type 1 diabetes mellitus Genes and Immunity. 2002;3: 235–249.

83. **Keisuke Ishii, Koichi Takakuwa, Takuya Mitsui and Kenichi Tanaka.** Studies on the human leukocyte antigen-DR in patients with endometriosis: genotyping of HLA-DRB1 alleles. Hum. Reprod 2002; 17 (3): 560-563.

84. Bischoff F, Simpson JL. Genetic basis of endometriosis. Ann N Y Acad Sci. 2004;1034: 284-99.

85. Baranova H., Botorishvilli R., Canis M., et al. Glutathioe S-transferase M1 gene polymorphism and susceptibility to endometriosis in a French population. Mol Hum Reprod 1997; 3:775-80.

86. Baranov V.S., Ivaschenko T., Bakay B.., et al. Proportion of the GSTM1 0/0 phenotype in some Slavic populations and its correlation with cystic fibrosis and some multifactorial diseases. Hum Genet 1996; 97:516-20).

87. Sun-Wei Guo. Glutathione S-transferases M1/T1 gene polymorphisms and endometriosis: a meta-analysis of genetic association studies Mol. Hum. Reprod 2005;11 (10): 729-743.

88. Cramer DW, Hornstein MD, Ng WG, Barbieri RL. Endometriosis associated with the N314D mutation of galactose-1-phosphate uridyl transferase (GALT). Mol Hum Reprod. 1996; 2(3):149-52.

89. Mayumi Morizane, Shigeki Yoshida, Satoshi Nakago, Shinya HamanaTakeshi Maruo, Stephen Kennedy, No Association of Endometriosis With Glutathione S-Transferase M1 and T1 Null Mutations in a Japanese Population Reproductive Sciences. 2004; 11(2): 118-121

90. Rai P, Kota V, Deendayal M, Shivaji S. Differential proteome profiling of eutopic endometrium from women with endometriosis to

understand etiology of endometriosis. J Proteome Res. 2010; 9(9):4407-19.

91. A.G. Braundmeier and A.T. Fazleabas. The non-human primate model of endometriosis: research and implications for fecundityMol. Hum. Reprod 2009;15 (10): 577-586.

92. Armstrong PB, Quigley JP and Sidebottom E. Transepithelial invasion and intramesenchymal infiltration of the chick embryo chorioallantois by tumor cell lines. Cancer Res 1982; 42, 1826–1837.

93. Malik E, Meyhofer-Malik A, Berg C, Bohm W, Kunzi-Rapp K, Diedrich K and Ruck A. Fluorescence diagnosis of endometriosis on the chorioallantoic membrane using 5-aminolaevulinic acid. Hum Reprod 2000; 15,584–588.

94. Maas JW, Groothuis PG, Dunselman GA, de Goeij AF, Struijker-Boudier HA and Evers JL. Development of endometriosis-like lesions after transplantation of human endometrial fragments onto the chick embryo chorioallantoic membrane. Hum Reprod 2001; 16,627–631.

95. Götte, M., Wolf, M., Staebler, A., Buchweitz, O., Kelsch, R., Schüring, A. and Kiesel, L. Increased expression of the adult stem cell marker Musashi-1 in endometriosis and endometrial carcinoma. The Journal of Pathology 2008; 215: 317–329.

96. Christopher L. Coe, Andrine M. Lemieux, Sherry E. Rier, Hideo Uno, and Michele L. Zimbric. Profile of Endometriosis in the Aging Female Rhesus MonkeyJ Gerontol A Biol Sci Med Sci 1998; 53A (1): M3-M7.

97. D'Hooghe TM, Bambra CS, Raeymaekers BM, Koninckx PR. Development of spontaneous endometriosis in baboons. Obstet Gynecol. 1996; 88(3):462-6.

98. Sherry E. Rier, Dan C. Martin, Robert E. Bowman, W. Paul Dmowski and Jeanne L. Becker. Endometriosis in Rhesus Monkeys (Macaca mulatta) Following Chronic Exposure to 2,3,7,8-Tetrachlorodibenzo-p-dioxin. Toxicol. Sci. 1993; 21 (4): 433-441.

99. Linda C Giudice, Lee C Kao. Endometriosis. Lancet 2004; 364: 1789–99.

100. Fanton JW, Golden JG. Radiation-induced endometriosis in Maccaca mulatta. Radiat Res 1991; 126: 141–46.

101. Rier SE, Martin DC, Bowman RE, et al. Endometriosis in rhesus monkeys (Maccaca mulatta) following chronic exposure to 2,3,7,8 tetrachlorodibenzo-p-dioxin. Fundam Appl Toxicol 1993; 21: 431–41.

102. Koninckx PR, Braet P, Kennedy SH, et al. Dioxin pollution and endometriosis in Belgium. Hum Reprod 1994; 91001–02.

103. Pauwels A, Schepens PJ, D'Hooghe T, Delbeke L, Dhont M, Brouwer A, Weyler J. The risks of endometriosis and exposure to dioxins and polychlorinated biphenyls: a case-controlled study of infertile women. Hum Reprod 2001; 16: 2050–55.

104. Eskenazi B, Mocarelli P, Warner M, et al. Serum dioxin concentrations and endometriosis: a cohort study in Seveso, Italy. Environ Health Perspect 2002; 110: 629–34.

105. Myers JP, Guillette LJ Jr, Palanza P, Parmigiani S, Swan SH, von Saal FS. The emerging science of endocrine disruption. Science and Culture Series. International Seminar on Nuclear War and Planetary Emergencies. 28th Session, 2003, Erice, Italy.

106. Sharpe RM, Franks S. Environment, lifestyle and infertility—an inter-generational issue. Nat Med 2002; suppl 8: s33–40.

107. Welshons WV, Thayer KA, Judy BM, Taylor JA, Curran EM, von Saal FS. Large effects from small exposures, I: mechanisms for endocrine disrupting chemicals with estrogen activity. Environ Health Perspect 2003; 222: 994–1006

108. Fjerbaek, A. and U.B. Knudsen, Endometriosis, dysmenorrhea and diet--what is the evidence? Eur J Obstet Gynecol Reprod Biol 2007; 132(2): 140-7.

109. Parazzini, F., et al., Selected food intake and risk of endometriosis. Hum Reprod 2004;19(8): 1755-9.

110. Heilier, J.F., et al., Environmental and host-associated risk factors in endometriosis and deep endometriotic nodules: a matched case-control study. Environ Res 2007; 103(1): 121-9.

111. Caserta, D., et al., Impact of endocrine disruptor chemicals in gynaecology. Hum Reprod Update 2008. 14(1): 59-72.

112. Arisawa, K., H. Takeda, and H. Mikasa, Background exposure to PCDDs/PCDFs/PCBs and its potential health effects: a review of epidemiologic studies. J Med Invest 2005; 52(1-2): 10-21.

113. Rier, S.E., et al., Endometriosis in rhesus monkeys (Macaca mulatta) following chronic exposure to 2,3,7,8-tetrachlorodibenzo-p-dioxin. Fundam Appl Toxicol 1993; 21(4): 433-41.

114. Arnold, D.L., et al., Prevalence of endometriosis in rhesus (Macaca mulatta) monkeys ingesting PCB (Aroclor 1254): review and evaluation. Fundam Appl Toxicol 1996; 31(1): 42-55.

115. Yang, J.Z., S.K. Agarwal, and W.G. Foster, Subchronic exposure to 2,3,7,8-tetrachlorodibenzo-p-dioxin modulates the pathophysiology of endometriosis in the cynomolgus monkey. Toxicol Sci, 2000; 56(2): 374-81.

116. Guo, S.W., The link between exposure to dioxin and endometriosis: a critical reappraisal of primate data. Gynecol Obstet Invest 2004; 57(3):157-73.

117. (WHO), W.H.O., Level of PCB's, PCDD's and PCDF's in breast milk: result of WHO coordinated inter-laboratory quality control studies and analytical field studies. WHO Environmental Health Series, 1989.

118. Eskenazi, B., et al., Serum dioxin concentrations and endometriosis: a cohort study in Seveso, Italy. Environ Health Perspect 2002; 110(7): 629-34.

119. Porpora, M.G., et al., Increased levels of polychlorobiphenyls in Italian women with endometriosis. Chemosphere 2006. 63(8): 1361-7.

120. Heilier, J.F., et al., Increased dioxin-like compounds in the serum of women with peritoneal endometriosis and deep endometriotic (adenomyotic) nodules. Fertil Steril 2005; 84(2): 305-12.

121. Cobellis, L., et al., Measurement of bisphenol A and bisphenol B levels in human blood sera from healthy and endometriotic women. Biomed Chromatogr, 2009.

122. Matthew David Rosser. The Emerging Role of Epigenetics in the Aetiology of Endometriosis. MSc thesis/ De Montfort University

123. Degen GH, Bolt HM. Endocrine disruptors: update on xenoestrogens. Int Arch Occup Environ Health. 2000; 73(7):433-41.

124. Morsch DM, Carneiro MM, Lecke SB, Araújo FC, Camargos AF, Reis FM, Spritzer PM. c-fos gene and protein expression in pelvic endometriosis: a local marker of estrogen action. J Mol Histol. 2009;40(1):53-8.

125. R Steinmetz,et al. N A Mitchner, A Grant, D L Allen, R M Bigsby, N Ben-Jonathan The xenoestrogen bisphenol A induces growth, differentiation, and c-fos gene expression in the female reproductive tract. Endocrinology 1998; 139 (6) : 2741-2747.

126. Hidekuni Inadera. The immune system as a target for environmental chemicals: Xenoestrogens and other compounds. Toxicology Letters 2008; 164 (3): 191-206.

4 CLINICAL ASPECTS OF ENDOMETRIOSIS

Clinical Presentations:

There are no sufficiently sensitive and specific signs and symptoms nor diagnostic tests for the clinical diagnosis of endometriosis. The clinical presentation is variable, with some women experiencing severe symptoms while others remain asymptomatic [2]. As there is a lack of pathognomonic symptoms and no useful noninvasive clinical tests to diagnose symptomatic disease are available, a delay in the diagnosis that averages from five to 11 years is observed [1, 3].

Common elements in the history include nulliparity and regular menstrual cycles with prolonged flow of 8 or more days. Onset of pain usually precedes flow by a few days and begins to resolve 1-2 days into the menses. Symptoms also usually improve during pregnancy and after menopause; they can recur postpartum or with postmenopausal hormone replacement therapy. A familial/genetic predisposition has been documented [4]. A woman with a first-degree relative with endometriosis has a lifetime risk of the disease approximately 10 times that of a woman without an affected family member. When the products of cyclic sloughing of endometriotic implants become entrapped by cyst formation, the resulting mass is referred to as an endometrioma. These can occur in any location but are most commonly found involving one or both ovaries. These masses can become quite painful, and patients with rupture present with an acute surgical abdomen [4].

Endometriosis should be considered in any woman of reproductive age who has pelvic pain. The most common symptoms are dysmenorrhea, dyspareunia, and lower back pain that worsens during menses [5-6]. Depending on the location of the implants, rectal pain and painful defecation may also occur. The diagnosis of endometriosis should be considered especially if a patient develops dysmenorrhea after years of pain-free menstrual cycles. Infertility may also be the presenting complaint. Infertile patients often have no painful symptoms, and their disease is only discovered in the course of the diagnostic work-up for infertility. The reason for this divergence in clinical manifestations is unknown [5,7].

Although a significant number of women with endometriosis remain asymptomatic (approximately one third) [4, 8], and the degree of visible endometriosis has no correlation with the degree of pain or other symptomatic impairment, because the location and depth of endometrial implants affect the symptoms [9]. However, pain does correlate with the depth of tissue infiltration, as pain is thought to be related to the degree of peritoneal inflammation rather than the volume of implants [10-11]. Symptoms of endometriosis can be variable but typically reflect the area of involvement. Such symptoms may include; dysmenorrheal, heavy or irregular bleeding, pelvic pain, lower abdominal or back pain, dyspareunia, pain on defecation often with cycles of diarrhea and constipation, bloating, nausea, vomiting, inguinal pain, pain on micturition and/or urinary frequency, and pain during exercise [4].

Endometriosis usually becomes apparent in the reproductive years when the lesions are stimulated by ovarian hormones. Symptoms tend to be strongest premenstrually, subsiding after cessation of menses [12]. A patient survey of women in the United Kingdom and United States who were referred to university- based endometriosis centers found that 70 to 71 percent presented with pelvic pain, 71 to 76 percent with dysmenorrhea, 44 percent with dyspareunia, and 15 to 20 percent with infertility [12-13]. In a British study of women with pelvic pain, many patients who eventually were diagnosed with endometriosis had been diagnosed previously with irritable bowel syndrome [14]. Endometriosis is associated with infertility because of adhesions that distort the pelvic anatomy and cause impaired ovum release and pickup. However, tubal distortion is not the only cause of infertility, because patients with endometriosis seem to have poor ovarian reserve with low oocyte and embryo quality [12]. A meta-analysis of 22 studies evaluating in vitro fertilization outcomes found that patients with endometriosis had a pregnancy rate of nearly one half that of patients without endometriosis, with decreases in fertilization, implantation, and oocyte production rates. [12, 15]

The patient usually presents with a history of progressively increasing pelvic pain and/or secondary dysmenorrheal since most endometriotic implants are found on the uterus, ovaries, and posterior peritoneum. Likewise, dysuria, flank pain, or hematuria may be present if the bladder or ureters are involved [4].

Cyclic pain is pain that accompanies bleeding at the time of menstruation. This could involve the bladder (hematuria), bowel (hematochezia and painful defecation), or, rarely, bleeding at uncommon sites such as the umbilicus, abdominal wall, or perineum [4]. A study reported that secondary dysmenorrhea occurs twice as often in women with endometriosis as in controls [16]. Pain frequently commences before menses. Endometriosis should be considered in a patient presenting with significant dysmenorrheal [4].

Patients who are sexually active may report deep dyspareunia that is worst in the premenstrual phase of the cycle. Deep dyspareunia may be due to scarring of the uterosacral ligaments, nodularity of the rectovaginal septum, and/or uterine retroversion, all of which may also lead to chronic backache. These symptoms are exaggerated during menses. Women with deep infiltration of the uterosacral ligaments were shown to have the most severe impairment of sexual function [17].

More uncommon cyclic symptoms include hemoptysis (pulmonary involvement), catamenial seizures (endometriotic lesions in the brain), and umbilical bleeding (implants in the umbilicus). Partial or complete bowel obstruction occasionally occurs because of either adhesion formation or a circumferential endometriosis lesion. Ureteral obstruction and hydronephrosis can result from endometrial implants on the ureter or mass effect from an endometrioma [4].

Pelvic pain which is the most common symptoms of endometriosis often correlates to the menstrual cycle, before and during menstruation and during ovulation. Women may also experience pelvic pain that doesn't correlate to their cycle or ovulation such as when passing urine, during sexual intercourse and in the lower back region. This is one of the reasons this condition is so unpredictable and frustrating [18]. For many women, the pain of endometriosis is so severe and debilitating that it impacts their lives in significant ways. Other symptoms that correlate with menstration are pain in the bowel, diarrhea or constipation, abdominal bloating and migraines. Women may also experience heavy or irregular bleeding, fatigue, irrital bowel syndrome, interstitial cystitis, fibromyalgia and infertility [18]. Endometriosis can cause scar tissue and adhesions to develop that can distort a woman's internal anatomy. In advanced stages, internal organs may fuse together, causing a condition known as frozen pelvis. This condition is not common, but is possible [18].

Dysmenorrhea was the chief complaint, reported by 62% of women with mainly peritoneal endometriosis in a Brazilian study [19-20]. In the same study, the prevalence of chronic pelvic pain was 57%, deep dyspareunia 55%, cyclic intestinal complaints 48%, infertility 40% and incapacitating dysmenorrhea 28%. [20]

The symptoms of endometriosis depend on the location of the disease. Deep endometriosis of the posterior pelvis is associated with increased severity of dyschezia, in comparison to women with pelvic endometriosis without posterior deep endometriosis [21]. Deep endometriosis of the rectovaginal septum is associated with the most severe forms of dyschezia and dyspareunia [21-22].

Intestinal complaints (periodic bloating, diarrhea or constipation) are some of the unrecognized symptoms of endometriosis [19-20, 23-24].

In a prospective, controlled study, cyclic bloating was seen in 96%, diarrhea in 27% and constipation in 16% of the women with endometriosis [24]. The corresponding numbers in women with no endometriosis were 64, 9 and 0%, respectively [19].

Adolescent women with endometriosis report a high rate of symptoms. Uterine cramping has been reported by 100%, cyclic pain 67%, non-cyclic pain 39%, constipation/diarrhea 67%, and referred pain (legs, back) by 31% of adolescents with laparoscopically diagnosed endometriosis [23].

Among infertile women undergoing laparoscopy, dysmenorrhea was the only symptom significantly predictive of endometriosis [25]. However, no differences in the rates of pelvic pain, dyspareunia or vaginal discharge were seen among women with endometriosis, compared to those with normal pelvis or adhesions [19, 25].

In a large retrospective analysis of the UK general practice research database concerning the prevalent symptoms within 3 years before the diagnosis of endometriosis [n=5540, each matched (year-of-birth and practice) to four controls], women with subsequent diagnosis of endometriosis had higher proportions of abdominopelvic pain or heavy menstrual bleeding (73 vs. 20%) [26]. When compared with controls, women with endometriosis had odds ratios [OR (95% CI)] for the following symptoms: abdominopelvic pain 5.2 (4.7–5.7), dysmenorrhea

8.1 (7.2–9.3), heavy menstrual bleeding 4.0 (3.5–4.5), infertility 8.2 (6.9–9.9), dyspareunia/postcoital bleeding 6.8 (5.7–8.2) and urinary tract symptoms 1.2 (1.0–1.3). In addition, history of diagnosis with ovarian cyst 7.3 (5.7–9.4), irritable bowel syndrome 1.6 (1.3–1.8), pelvic inflammatory disease 3.0 (2.5-3.6) and fibrocystic breast disease 1.4 (1.2–1.7) were risk factors for subsequent diagnosis of endometriosis. Increasing the number of symptoms increased the chance of having endometriosis. In addition, women with eventual diagnosis endometriosis had consulted the doctor more frequently, and were twice as likely to have had time off from work [19,26].

In the same study, women with endometriosis had a high incidence of having received a diagnosis of irritable bowel syndrome: OR (95% CI) for irritable bowel syndrome 3.5 (3.1–3.9) before and 2.5 (2.2–2.8) after the diagnosis of endometriosis. In addition, the incidence of having received the diagnosis of pelvic inflammatory disease is higher among women with endometriosis. In the UK general practice research database study the OR (95% CI) of pelvic inflammatory disease diagnosis was 5.9 (5.1–6.9) before and 3.8 (5.1–6.9) after the diagnosis of endometriosis [19, 26].

In an Italian study, women scheduled to undergo various gynaecological operations were interviewed concerning infertility, dysmenorrhea, dyspareunia and non-cyclical pelvic pain. None of these was predictive of the diagnosis of endometriosis [27]. However, women eventually surgically diagnosed with endometriosis reported more intensive dysmenorrhea than those with no diagnosis of endometriosis [19, 27-28].

Physical Examination

Physical examination in endometriosis is aimed at facilitating diagnosis and treatment of the disease. Patients with endometriosis do not frequently have any physical findings beyond tenderness related to the site of involvement [29-31]. The most common finding is nonspecific pelvic tenderness. In one study, 22% of adolescents had abnormal physical findings consistent with anatomic lesions found during surgery [4].

On pelvic evaluation, tenderness upon examination is best detected at the time of menses. The hallmark finding on examination is the presence of tender nodular masses along thickened uterosacral ligaments, the posterior uterus, or the posterior cul-de-sac [4]. Obliteration of the cul-de-sac in conjunction with fixed uterine retroversion implies extensive disease. Occasionally, a bluish nodule may be seen in the vagina due to infiltration from the posterior vaginal wall. Rupture of an ovarian endometrioma may present as an acute abdomen [4]. Extensive involvement of the rectum and other areas of the gastrointestinal (GI) tract may cause adhesions and obstruction. Examination should also include evaluation for cervicitis, abnormal discharge, and sexually transmitted diseases (STDs) [4].

Clinical examination in endometriosis includes inspection of the vagina using a speculum as well as bimanual and rectovaginal palpation [19,32]. Clinical examination in women suspected with endometriosis includes physical examination of the pelvis but also the inspection and palpation of the abdomen. Location and extent of disease can sometimes be determined by clinical examination [19, 32].

There should be special emphasis on the visualization of deep endometriosis in the vagina by inspection of the posterior fornix of the vaginal wall [32].

Vaginal examination can facilitate the detection of infiltration or nodules of the vagina, uterosacral ligaments or pouch of Douglas [32]. Rectovaginal digital examination may allow the detection of infiltration or mass involving the rectosigmoidal colon or adnexal masses [19, 27, 32].

A prospective study has demonstrated that reliability of the clinical examination in detecting pelvic endometriosis is improved during menstruation [33]. However, overall, the evidence on the value of clinical examination for the diagnosis of endometriosis is weak, mainly based on cohort studies [19].

Staging:

Staging the disorder helps physicians formulate a treatment plan and evaluate response to therapy. According to Revised Classification of the American Society of Reproductive Medicine stated 4 stages of endometriosis [34], based on number, location, and depth of implants and presence of filmy or dense adhesions. These are:

Stage I (Minimal): Findings restricted to only superficial lesions and possibly a few filmy adhesions.

Stage II (Mild): In addition, some deep lesions are present in the cul-de-sac.

Stage III (Moderate): As above, plus presence of endometriomas on the ovary and more adhesions.

Stage IV (Severe): As above, plus large endometriomas, extensive adhesions.

Endometrioma on the ovary of any significant size (Approx. 2 cm +) must be removed surgically because hormonal treatment alone will not remove the full endometrioma cyst, which can progress to acute pain from the rupturing of the cyst and internal bleeding. Endometrioma is sometimes misdiagnosed as ovarian cysts. Moderate and severe endometriosis are characterized by chocolate cysts and severe adhesions. The stage of endometriosis does not necessarily reflect the level of pain, risk of infertility or symptoms present. For example, it is possible for a woman in Stage I to be in an abundant amount pain, while a woman in Stage IV may be asymptomatic. "In addition, women who receive treatment during the first two stages of the disease have the greatest chance of regaining their ability to become pregnant following treatment.

This classification is a fairly accurate method of recording laparoscopic findings. However, high intraobserver and interobserver variability precludes its use in comparing the outcomes of therapeutic studies [35]. Furthermore, this staging system does not correlate well with pain and dyspareunia [36], and fecundity rates cannot be predicted accurately [4].

However, the patient's stage is useful in determining her prognosis for subsequent reproduction. The staging system can also be used to monitor a patient's response to therapeutic efforts. Surgical exploration is required for this staging system, both initially and for subsequent follow-up [4].

Attempts to develop a staging system that meets the need to establish a common language in endometriosis surgical findings, enable specificity of diagnosis, standardize comparisons, and facilitate research have been undertaken. Adamson and Pasta *[37],* have subsequently developed a validated, clinically useful tool for surgically confirmed patients with endometriosis attempting non-IVF conception

Differential Diagnosis

Given the nonspecific symptoms of endometriosis, the differential diagnosis is lengthy [12, 38]. The possibility of malignancy must be considered.

Differential diagnosis of endometriosis by symptoms regarding secondary dysmenorrhea may be caused by adenomyosis, myomas, infection, and cervical stenosis, while causes of dyspareunia should be excluded like diminished lubrication or vaginal expansion, because of insufficient arousal, gastrointestinal causes (e.g., constipation, irritable bowel syndrome), infection, musculoskeletal causes (e.g., pelvic relaxation, levator spasm), pelvic vascular congestion, urinary causes (e.g., urethral syndrome, interstitial cystitis). While regarding generalized pelvic pain causes should be excluded like endometritis, neoplasms, benign or malignant, nongynecologic causes, ovarian torsion, pelvic adhesions, pelvic inflammatory disease, and sexual or physical abuse. However, regarding presence of infertility other causes should be excluded like anovulation, cervical factors (e.g., mucus, sperm, antibodies, stenosis), luteal phase deficiency, male factor infertility, and Tubal disease or infection [12, 38]. Hence, the differential diagnosis is large as endometriosis can mimic many other conditions such as pelvic inflammatory disease, cervicitis, benign or malignant ovarian masses, pelvic adhesions, urinary tract infections, interstitial cystitis, irritable bowel syndrome, constipation, and other anorectal disease. Generally speaking, the most common differential diagnosis are appendicitis, chlamydial genitourinary infections, diverticulitis, ectopic pregnancy, gonorrhea, ovarian cysts, ovarian torsion, pelvic inflammatory disease, and urinary tract Infection in females [4].

Complications:

A brief allusion to the likely complications of endometriosis merits mention in this context.

Complications of endometriosis embrace the following

- The bleeding can give rise to bands of scar tissue with resultant adhesions to the organs in the pelvis and abdomen.

- Decrease fertility without any apparent cause or may be due to adhesions forming on or near to the ovaries or fallopian tubes.

- An augmented danger of miscarriage or premature delivery..

- Bleeding may occur from cysts synchronous with normal menstruation

- At this juncture it is pertinent to refer to the case reported by Harmanli et al [39]. This was an exceptional case of massive hemoperitoneum due to bleeding from a tubal endometriosis implant in a previously healthy 29-year-old woman without prior history of endometriosis [39]. Idrees [40], has described a 41-year-old woman with prior history of breast carcinoma who had bilateral salpingo-oophorectomy because of hematosalpinx [40].

- Rupture of the cyst with or without haemorrhage causing severe pain.

- Endometriosis of appendix presenting as acute appendicitis has been reported . The incidence of appendiceal endometriosis is 2.8%. Oulaqi *et al* [41], have reported the case of a 25-year-old woman who was diagnosed as acute appendicitis associated with primary infertility had histopathological confirmnation of endmetriosis of appendix.[41-42]. Perforation of the appendix may occur especially during the first two trimesters of pregnancy.

- A case of endometriosis with massive ascites has been on record [43].

- An augmented hazard of certain types of cancer, especially ovarian. In this context we shall briefly refer the malignant potential of endometriosis

References

1. Márcia Mendonça Carneiro, Ivone Dirk de Sousa Filogônio, Luciana Maria Pyramo Costa, Ivete de Ávila, andMárcia Cristina França Ferreira. Clinical Prediction of Deeply Infiltrating Endometriosis before Surgery: Is It Feasible? A Review of the Literature, BioMed Research International, Hindawi Publishing Corporation, 2013, Article ID 564153, 8 pages.

2. A. A.Murphy. "Clinical aspects of endometriosis," Annals of the New York Academy of Sciences, 2002; 955: 1–10.

3. K. Ballard, K. Lowton, and J.Wright, "What's the delay?Aqualitative study of women's experiences of reaching a diagnosis of endometriosis," Fertility and Sterility 2006; 86 (5): 1296– 1301.

4. Dharmesh Kapoor, et al. Endometriosis Clinical Presentation.

Available at http://emedicine.medscape.com/article/271899-clinical. Accessed 20th March 2014.

5. Neha Agarwal and Arulselvi Subramanian. Endometriosis – Morphology, Clinical Presentations and Molecular Pathology. J Lab Physicians. 2010; 2(1): 1–9.

6. American College of Obstetricians and Gynecologists. Washington DC: ACOG; 1993. Endometriosis.ACOG technical bulletin no. 184.

7. Wellbery C. Diagnosis and treatment of endometriosis. Am Fam Physician. 1999;60:1753–68.

8. Buchweitz O, Poel T, Diedrich K, Malik E. The diagnostic dilemma of minimal and mild endometriosis under routine conditions. J Am Assoc Gynecol Laparosc. Feb 2003; 10(1):85-9.

9. Demco L. Mapping the source and character of pain due to endometriosis by patient-assisted laparoscopy. J Am Assoc Gynecol Laparosc 1998; 5(3):241-5.

10. Koninckx PR, Martin DC. Deep endometriosis: a consequence of infiltration or retraction or possibly adenomyosis externa?. Fertil Steril 1992; 58(5):924-8.

11. Koninckx PR, Oosterlynck D, D'Hooghe T, Meuleman C. Deeply infiltrating endometriosis is a disease whereas mild endometriosis could be considered a non-disease. Ann N Y Acad Sci. 1994; 734:333-41.

12. Anne L. Mounsey, Alex Wilgus, David C. Slawson. Diagnosis and Management of Endometriosis. American Family Physician, 2006; 74 (4). Available at www.aafp.org/afp. Downloaded 20th March 2014.

13. Kuohung W, Jones GL, Vitonis AF, Cramer DW, Kennedy SH, Thomas D, et al. Characteristics of patients with endometriosis in the United States and the United Kingdom. Fertil Steril 2002; 78:767-72.

14. Zondervan KT, Yudkin PL, Vessey MP, Dawes MG, Barlow DH, Kennedy SH. Patterns of diagnosis and referral in women consulting for chronic pelvic pain in UK primary care. Br J Obstet Gynaecol 1999; 106:1156-61.

15. Barnhart K, Dunsmoor-Su R, Coutifaris C. Effect of endometriosis on in vitro fertilization. Fertil Steril 2002; 77:1148-55.

16. Williams TJ, Pratt JH. Endometriosis in 1,000 consecutive celiotomies: incidence and management. Am J Obstet Gynecol 1977; 129(3):245-50.

17. Ferrero S, Esposito F, Abbamonte LH, Anserini P, Remorgida V, Ragni N. Quality of sex life in women with endometriosis and deep dyspareunia. Fertil Steril 2005;83(3):573-9.

18. Endometriosis. Available at http://endometriosis.org/ Accessed March 20, 2014.

19. Management of women with endometriosis. Guideline of the European Society of Human Reproduction and Embryology. ESHRE Endometriosis Guideline Development Group September 2013.

20. Bellelis P, Dias JA, Jr., Podgaec S, Gonzales M, Baracat EC and Abrão MS. Epidemiological and clinical aspects of pelvic endometriosis a case series. Rev Assoc Med Bras 2010; 56:467–471.

21. Seracchioli R, Mabrouk M, Guerrini M, Manuzzi L, Savelli L, Frascà C and Venturoli S. Dyschezia and posterior deep infiltrating endometriosis: analysis of 360 cases. J Minim Invasive Gynecol 2008; 15:695–699.

22. Thomassin I, Bazot M, Detchev R, Barranger E, Cortez A and Darai E. Symptoms before and after surgical removal of colorectal endometriosis that are assessed by magnetic resonance imaging and rectal endoscopic sonography. Am J Obstet Gynecol 2004; 190:1264–1271.

23. Davis GD, Thillet E and Lindemann J. Clinical characteristics of adolescent endometriosis. J Adolesc Health 1993; 14:362–368.

24. Luscombe GM, Markham R, Judio M, Grigoriu A and Fraser IS. Abdominal bloating: an under-recognized endometriosis symptom. J Obstet Gynaecol Can 2009; 31:1159–1171.

25. Forman RG, Robinson JN, Mehta Z and Barlow DH. Patient history as a simple predictor of pelvic pathology in subfertile women. Hum Reprod 1993; 8:53–55.

26. Ballard KD, Seaman HE, de Vries CS and Wright JT. Can symptomatology help in the diagnosis of endometriosis? Findings from a national case-control study—Part 1. BJOG 2008; 115:1382–1391.

27. Eskenazi B, Warner M, Bonsignore L, Olive D, Samuels S and Vercellini P. Validation study of nonsurgical diagnosis of endometriosis. Fertil Steril 2001; 76:929–935.

28. Hsu AL, Sinaii N, Segars J, Nieman LK and Stratton P. Relating pelvic pain location to surgical findings of endometriosis. Obstet Gynecol 2011; 118:223–230.

29. Mounsey AL, Wilgus A, Slawson DC. Diagnosis and management of endometriosis. Am Fam Physician 2006; 74(4):594-600.

30. Kennedy S, Bergqvist A, Chapron C, D'Hooghe T, Dunselman G, Greb R, et al. ESHRE guideline for the diagnosis and treatment of endometriosis. Hum Reprod 2005;20(10):2698-704.

31. Kingsberg SA, Janata JW. Female sexual disorders: assessment, diagnosis, and treatment. Urol Clin North Am 2007;34(4):497-506, v-vi.

32. Bazot M, Lafont C, Rouzier R, Roseau G, Thomassin-Naggara I and Daraï E. Diagnostic accuracy of physical examination, transvaginal sonography, rectal endoscopic sonography, and magnetic resonance imaging to diagnose deep infiltrating endometriosis. Fertil Sterll 2009; 92:1825–1833.

33. Koninckx PR, Meuleman C, Oosterlynck D and Cornillie FJ. Diagnosis of deep endometriosis by clinical examination during menstruation and plasma CA-125 concentration. Fertil Steril 1996; 65:280–287.

34. American Society For Reproductive M. "Revised American Society for Reproductive Medicine classification of endometriosis: 1996". Fertility and Sterility 1997; 67 (5): 817–21

35. Hornstein MD, Gleason RE, Orav J, Haas ST, Friedman AJ, Rein MS, et al. The reproducibility of the revised American Fertility Society classification of endometriosis. Fertil Steril. 1993; 59(5):1015-21.

36. Koninckx PR, Meuleman C, Demeyere S, Lesaffre E, Cornillie FJ. Suggestive evidence that pelvic endometriosis is a progressive disease, whereas deeply infiltrating endometriosis is associated with pelvic pain. Fertil Steril. Apr 1991; 55(4):759-65.

37. Adamson GD, Pasta DJ. Endometriosis fertility index: the new, validated endometriosis staging system. Fertil Steril. 2010; 94(5):1609-1615.

38. American College of Obstetrics and Gynecology. Chronic pelvic pain. ACOG technical bulletin no. 223. Washington, D.C.: American College of Obstetrics and Gynecology, 1996:3.

39. Harmanli OH, Chatwani A, Caya JG. Massive hemoperitoneum from endometriosis of the fallopian tube. A case report. J Reprod Med 1998; 43:716-8.

40. Idrees M, Zakashansky K, Kalir T. Xanthogranulomatous salpingitis associated with fallopian tube mucosal endometriosis: a clue to the pathogenesis. Ann Diagn Pathol 2007; 11:117-21.

41. Al Oulaqi NS, Hefny AF, Joshi S, Salim K, Abu-Zidan FM. Endometriosis of the appendix. Afr Health Sci 2008;8:196-8.

42. Gustofson RL, Kim N, Liu S, Stratton P. Endometriosis and the appendix: a case series and comprehensive review of the literature. Fertil Steril 2006;86:298-303.

43. Cheong EC, Lim DT. Massive ascites-an uncommon presentation of endometriosis. Singapore Med J 2003; 44:98-100.

5 EXTRAPELVIC ENDOMETRIOSIS

Endometrium is one of the most extraordinary tissues of the human body. The ability of endometrium to be implanted in different tissues and simultaneously to maintain its functionality is very impressive. It also explains the variety of symptoms that are components of endometriosis syndrome [1].

Cutaneous Endometriosis

Endometriosis uncommonly occurs in the abdominal wall and its occurrence in a post-operative scar is rare [2]. Blanco et al. [3] reported 10 cases of scar endometriosis of which 9 cases followed caesarean section and one occurred in laparotomy for ectopic pregnancy. Pathan et al, [4], described seven cases that occurred in caesarean and one occurred in a hysterectomy scar. Horton et al. [5] in their review of 445 cases of abdominal wall endometriosis recorded that 57, 11 and 12% cases occurred in scars of caesarean section, hysterectomy and other surgical procedures, respectively. Twenty percent cases occurred in other sites such as umbilicus and the groin.

Majority of abdominal wall endometriosis occur in or adjacent to surgical scars, subsequent to caesarean section or hysterectomy. Laparotomy scar endometriosis after salpingectomy for ectopic pregnancy has seldom been reported [6]. Zaheer et al., reported a case of scar endometriosis following laparotomy for chronic ectopic, and diagnosed by fine needle aspiration cytology (FNAC) which was further confirme excision biopsy [5]. Prof. Kannan Kutty from Malaysia have seen five cases of umbilical endometriois during the past thirty years (unpublished data). The clinical diagnosis in all these cases ranged from desmoid, umbilical hernia to fibrosarcoma and the diagnosis in all these cases were established by excision biopsy.

A case was reported that of a 46-year-old woman in whom endometriosis appeared as a cutaneous black mass in the umbilicus. Besides its infrequent occurrence its pathogenesis remains unclear [7].

One of the theories regarding the pathogenesis has been suggested: (1) the most favored metastatic theory states the transport of endometrial cells to adjacent locations via surgical manipulations, hematogenous or lymphatic dissemination and (2) primitive pluripotential mesenchymal cells undergo specialised differentiation and metaplasia into endometrial tissue (metaplastic theory) [8]. It is important to include endometriosis in the differential diagnosis of uncertain skin lesions of the umbilicus, even in cases with no previous abdominal surgery [6]. Furthermore umbilical endometriosis of the skin can have different appearances that simulate malignant tumors, and radical surgery with histology is therefore indicated.

It is supposed that the disease might stem from metaplasia of urachus remnants in case of isolated umbilical endometriosis [9]. Those patients commonly present with a brownish or bluish painful umbilical nodule, as noted in our patient. A few series have reported bleeding from the nodule. A slow-growing umbilical mass associated with cyclical pain during menstruation and brown color gives a picture clinically characteristic of cutaneous endometriosis [10].

Umbilical endometriosis of the skin can have different appearances that resemble malignant tumors, and radical surgery with histology is therefore indicated [7,11]. Three patients presented with primary isolated spontaneous umbilical endometriosis. One of them was having co-incidentally autosomal dominant polycystic disease of liver and kidneys. Another one was never pregnant and never had pelvic surgery which is very rare [7,12]. Razzi et al report a case of umbilical endometriosis in a pregnant woman at 16 weeks of gestation [7, 13].

Regarding pathogenesis of these cases; a physical transplantation of endometrial cells during surgery seems to be the most likely mechanism of development. However, cutaneous endometriosis can occur in women without a history of surgery, usually appearing in the umbilicus [14].

Cutaneous endometriosis also has occurred in women without intrapelvic endometriosis and without a history of symptoms suggestive of endometriosis. [14-16] The pathogenesis of such cases is even less clear. Proposed mechanisms include spread of existing endometrial cells via lymphatics or blood, or de novo development from pluripotent cells of the coelom [17-18]

The mean time to histologic diagnosis of cutaneous endometriosis is more than 2 years from symptom onset [19]. Classically, women found to have cutaneous endometriosis report a slowly enlarging nodule, with cyclic pain and bleeding at the site corresponding with menses. Even without these characteristic symptoms, cutaneous endometriosis should be considered in the differential diagnosis of an umbilical nodule. While the risk for malignant transformation of cutaneous endometriosis is very low, rare cases have been reported [20], making prompt diagnosis and subsequent surgical treatment important for preventing unnecessary morbidity and mortality [14].

Urinary Tract Endometriosis

Reports, rare though, of endometriosis of the urinary tract have appeared in the literature. Its reported incidence is between 0.01% and 1.2%. Involvement of the urinary tract at the vesical, ureteral or renal level ranges from 1% and 11% in a ratio of 40:5:1 [21], reflecting an overall rate of urinary tract involvement of 1%–2% of all cases [7, 22-25]. The ratio of bladder-to-ureteral-to-renal involvement is 40:5:1 [26-27]. Andrew feifer et al [28], have reported a case of obstructive uropathy linked with primnary endometrial ureteral endometrioma [28].

Endometriosis of kidney is a rare condition [1]. The common symptoms of renal endometriosis are local pain and rarely cyclical hematuria. It usually comes suddenly as a clinical manifestation. Sometimes the lesion may be totally asymptomatic and may diagnosed after nephrectomy for presumed renal cell carcinoma [29-30]. In ureteral endometriosis, ureteral involvement is often limited to one ureter, most commonly the left [1].

Two major pathological types exist: extrinsic and intrinsic ureteral endometriosis [1]. In the most common extrinsic type endometrial glandular and stromal tissue and the adventitia of the ureter or surrounding connective tissues are involved. In the intrinsic type muscularis propria, lamina propria, or ureteral lumen are involved [31-32]. Ureteral endometriosis can lead to urinary tract obstruction with subsequent hydroureter and hydronephrosis and even loss of renal function which is rare [1, 33].

Although ureteral and bladder endometriosis both occur in the urinary tract, they do not frequently coexist and their clinical presentation and management are different. Bladder endometriosis often mimicks recurrent cystitis, but rarely results in severe sequelae [34]. Ureteral endometriosis is often asymptomatic, but can lead to silent loss of renal function. Renal and urethral involvements are rare and only as case reports.The overall prevalence of urinary endometriosis is unclear but may occur in 1 -4% of all cases of endometriosis, however, in bladder is 70 – 80% of all urinary tract involvements, while involvement of ureter is about 15 – 20% of all urinary tract involvements, Kidney 4% of all urinary tract involvements, Urethra 2% of all urinary tract involvements [34].

Renal endometriosis is rarely encountered, it is briefly mentioned in the clinical guidelines and literatures, however, ureteral endometriosis may be involved in 15% to 20% of the urinary tract cases. Bilateral disease in ureter has been reported in up to 23% of cases. The left side is more often affected, which may be because the sigmoid colon prevents the regurgitated endometrial cells to be cleared by the peritoneal fluid on the left side.

Ureteral involvement may be either intrinsic or extrinsic. If endometrial glands and stroma are within the lamina propria, tunica muscularis, or ureteral lumen it is said Intrinsic endometriosis and if they are localized within periureteral tissue extrinsic endometriosis ensues

[34]. Eighty percent of ureteral endometriosis is extrinsic and most commonly involves the distal ureter. Differentiation between these two forms of ureteral endometriosis has histologic and pathogenetic importance, but has little impact on clinical management since the precise location of the lesion cannot be determined preoperatively. Moreover, both intrinsic and extrinsic forms of the disease may result in ureteral stenosis [34].

Silent loss of renal function has been reported in 25% to 43% of patients with ureteral endometriosis, which may result in total loss of function of the affected kidney. Historically, up to one third of kidneys affected by ureteral endometriosis were lost. So, it has been recommended to take image of the upper urinary tract in all patients with pelvic endometriosis with ultrasonography or IVU [34].

Bladder endometriosis is defined as the presence of endometrial glands and stroma at detrusor muscle. Bladder endometriosis causes nonspecific urinary symptoms, including urinary frequency, urgency, dysuria, or urinary retention. Occurrence of these symptoms during menses is suggestive. Cyclic hematuria is uncommon but characteristic. The ureteral openings are usually not involved by the vesical lesions so, hydronephrosis is rare. Some women with bladder endometriosis are asymptomatic and present with an incidental finding of a bladder nodule on pelvic imaging or as a result of pelvic surgery. Some patients are asymptomatic for the first few years and will only realize that they have the disease when it is already in its serious stage, manifesting more severe symptoms. The most common complaint of women that have bladder endometriosis is pain in the abdominal or pelvic area. The degree of pain can be mild to severe or acute to subacute. Usually, this pain will be more intense during monthly period. Women with bladder endometriosis also experience various urinary problems [34].

Endometriosis of Gastrointestinal Tract

Endometriotic implants of the gastrointestinal tract are estimated to occur in 12-37% of patients with endometriosis [7, 35]. It most commonly affects those segments of bowel in the dependent portion of the pelvis and is rarely found proximal to the terminal ileum [36]. The most commonly affected areas in decreasing order of frequency are the rectosigmoid colon, appendix, cecum, and distal ileum [36-37]. The implants are usually serosal but can eventually erode through the subserosal layers and cause marked thickening and fibrosis of the muscularis propria. An intact overlying mucosa is almost always present, since the implanted tissue only rarely invades through to the mucosa [36]. Inflammatory response to cyclic hemorrhage can lead to adhesions, bowel stricture, and gastrointestinal obstruction [7].

Goldsmith *et al* report a case of hepatic endometriosis in a postmenopausal woman who presented with right upper quadrant pain as her only symptom [38]. There have only been 11 previously reported cases of hepatic endometrioma [7]. Lee, 2009 [39] reviewed the clinicopathologic findings of 18 samples from 15 patients with intestinal endometriosis. Three cases were associated with adenocarcinoma in the same or different segments; specifically, two primary rectal adenocarcinomas and one endometrioid adenocarcinoma arising from endometriosis [7, 39].

Oulaqi et al have reported the case of a 25-year-old woman who was admitted with a diagnosis of acute appendicitis associated with primary infertility. Histopathological examination of the appendix revealed endometriosis [40]. The prevalence of appendiceal endometriosis is 2.8%. [41]. Involvement of the appendix may present as appendicitis, mucocele of appendix, or appendicular mass that may mimic a neoplasm. Perforation of the appendix may occur especially during the first two trimesters of pregnancy [7, 42-43].

The common endometriosis bowel symptoms are the rectal bleeding and pain, the painful bowel movements, the loss of appetite, the cramping stomach pains, the nausea and vomiting, the constipation and/ or diarrhea, the abdominal bloating and gas in the abdomen. All these symptoms are getting worse during menstruation [1, 44-47].

The most common location of extrapelvic intestinal endometriosis is the last part of the ileum (the small intestine), the cecum (the first part of the large bowel), and the appendix [1, 48].

Endometriosis can also be located in the liver and the gallbladder, but these entities are extremely rare [1]. There are approximately fourteen cases in the international literature about liver endometriosis and in most of them the patients were suffering from pain and a feeling of weight in the right upper quadrant of the abdomen [1].

There are also cases of liver endometriosis that was present with the clinical expression of obstructive jaundice [49--53].

Endometriosis of the gallbladder is extremely rare. There are two case reports in the literature referring to the diagnosis of gallbladder endometriosis [1, 54].

Lia C, et al 2011 [55], have recorded 89 patients from a single institution with histologically confirmed, symptomatic intestinal endometriosis from 1 January 1994 to 30 September 2009 and reviewed these cases. Abdominal pain was the most common symptom in patients with intestinal endometriosis; however, rectal bleeding was significantly associated with intestinal endometriosis of the distal colon, while dysfunctional uterine bleeding was seen more in patients with proximal intestinal endometriosis. Preoperative confirmation of intestinal endometriosis was uncommon; colonoscopy with biopsy confirmed the diagnosis in 29.6 % of patients tested and only 15 % of patients with intestinal endometriosis had histologic lesions involving mucosa. In the five patients who underwent endoscopic ultrasound (EUS), the diagnosis of intestinal endometriosis was established in all cases ($n = 4$) where histology or cytology was obtained. Malignancy was considered nearly as frequently as intestinal endometriosis preoperatively, and 90.4 % of patients underwent laparotomy as the initial surgical approach [55]. They concluded that intestinal endometriosis can present with a variety of manifestations, which may provide clues to location of bowel affected. Patients with known pelvic endometriosis and rectal bleeding are more likely to have distal bowel affected. Making a diagnosis of intestinal endometriosis preoperatively may allow for less invasive surgical approaches and better patient outcomes [55].

Yu-Hung Lin, et al 2006 [56] have presented an unusual case of intestinal endometriosis in general surgical practice. They concluded that it is difficult to make a definite diagnosis of endometriosis with bowel involvement before surgery [56]. It should be considered in any premenopausal woman who complains of gastrointestinal symptoms, especially when the patient has cyclic symptoms with a history of endometriosis [56]. The severity of an obstructive symptom could be helpful for the choice of surgery or hormone therapy. Those with a history of hormonal replacement therapy or a postmenopausal status should be treated more carefully against the higher possibility of malignancy. Laparoscopy should be used for the diagnosis of endometriosis and may be considered for treatment by skilled surgeons [56].

The diagnosis of intestinal endometriosis should be considered in any premenopausal woman who complains of gastrointestinal symptoms, especially when there are cyclic symptoms and a history of endometriosis [56- 59]. However, most cases are found accidentally from surgery. Imaging studies such as CT and MRI are not sensitive enough for definite diagnosis, with only about 70% sensitivity and specificity [60]. Colonoscopic biopsy rarely yields the diagnosis, since the endometriosis is usually located subserosally [59]. Laparoscopy remains the only investigation able to confirm the presence of intestinal endometriosis prior to laparotomy [56-57].

Suhar Al-Saad et al 2007 [61] have reviewed six patients with extra-gonadal endometriosis who presented to the surgical department in Bahrain Kingdom during a period of three years (between 2002 –2005). They reported that primary endometriosis of the appendix could be accompanied with ovarian cyst which was histologically diagnosed as a teratoma [61]. Appendiceal endometriosis, while relatively uncommon in patients with endometriosis, it is rare in the general population. In patients with right lower quadrant or pelvic pain, the appendix should be inspected for endometriosis and any evidence of nongynecologic disease [62]. Same study [61] reviewed a patient who presented with acute small bowel obstruction secondary to primary endometriosis [61]. This is similar to a case was reported of a young Nigerian female diagnosed with chronic intestinal obstruction due to rectosigmoid endometriosis causing stricture. She was successfully treated [63]. Another case presented was a pre-menopausal woman with severe constipation causing intermittent obstruction [61]. Colonoscopy revealed a tight rectal stricture; however, mucosal biopsies were normal. Exploratory surgery revealed an intense fibrotic reaction involving the rectum and uterus, necessitating a simultaneous low anterior resection and hysterectomy. Pathology established a diagnosis of endometriosis [64]. The pre-operative diagnosis of rectal endometriosis can be difficult to establish. Endometrial deposits do not invade the mucosa; therefore, colonoscopy with biopsies is non-diagnostic [61]. Surgery may be the only definitive way to obtain the diagnosis. Rectal endometriosis must be included in the differential diagnosis of rectal stricture [61, 64].

Thoracic Endometriosis

Endometriosis of the lung is associated with catamenial hemoptysis and chest pain. It is rare, chronic, and estrogen dependent [65]. Confirmation requires a combination of clinical symptoms and postoperative histopathological assessment [66]. Clinical examination often reveals only occult symptoms and signs, but severe cases can result in extensive decidual adhesions and distortion of tissue in the proximity of the decidua. It is these that lead to catamenial pain and hemoptysis, and the disease can be suspected in women with these symptoms [67].

The pathologist's role is made additionally difficult by the disease's

many histologic features, from typical endometrial glands to an

abundance of fibrous tissue [66].

For women with lung endometriosis, surgery is able to provide

radical relief. Because of the high rate of recrudescence, surgical salvage

may be expected [68]. Medical therapies have historically included

administration of contraceptive progestogens, gonadotropin-releasing

hormone agonists, androgens, and non-steroidal anti-inflammatory

drugs. Treatments to lower circulating estradiol concentrations may be

useful for only a limited time due to unacceptable side effects, and

changes or additional medications are commonly needed [66, 69].

There are three main theories of pathogenesis for thoracic

endometriosis [7, 70-74]. Sampson theorized that menstrual blood with

endometrial fragments could regurgitate from fallopian tube into

peritoneal cavity. This blood could find its way to the subphrenic space

and pass through the diaphragmatic fenestrations to the pleural cavity.

Ivanoff theorized that irritant blood with endometrial fragments could

pass through such fenestrations and produce metaplasia of pleural

surface which is histologically similar to that of peritoneum. However

these two theories do not explain parenchymal disease. Some theorize

that obstetrical and gynecological procedures that disrupt endometrial

blood vessels and lymphatics may allow lymphovascular entry of endometrial tissue causing parenchymal disease [7]. This observation is linked with common association of pulmonary endometriosis and certain forms of endometrial trauma. A presumptive diagnosis of pulmonary endometriosis can be made with a typical clinical history. Yusuf reports a case of pleural endometriosis in a 28 years infertile lady who presented with catamenial hemothorax occurring in the first 3 days of menstruation over a 3 months period associated with right shoulder pain and progressive shortness of breath for last 6 years [7, 74]. Agrawal et al 2009 [75], have reported a case of 47-year-old woman who had undergone hysterectomy and bilateral salpingo-oophorectomy for endometriosis and presented 4 years after surgery with a well-differentiated endometrioid adenocarcinoma arising in the background of endometriosis in the right chest wall [7, 75].

Huang et al., 2013 [65], reported a case of endometriosis of the lung in a 29-year-old woman with long-term periodic catamenial hemoptysis. In this patient a chest computed tomography image obtained during menstruation revealed a radiographic opaque lesion in the lingular segment of the left superior lobe.. During bronchoscopy, bleeding in the mucosa of the distal bronchus of the lingular segment of the left superior lobe was observed. Histopathology subsequent to an exploratory thoracotomy confirmed the diagnosis of endometriosis of the left lung [65].

The clinical symptom of thoracic endometriosis, as is hematothorax and pneumothorax. Menstruation related hemoptysis is not obviously present in all patients, and accurate diagnosis of thoracic endometriosis is always difficult to make [65]. Huang et al., 2013 [65] reviewed 74 cases of catamenial hemoptysis that have been reported since 1956 [76] in which ectopic endometriosis was identified: 37 cases were in the right lung, 19 in the left, and 6 were bilateral. In 61 of 70 patients (87.1%) who underwent gynecological examinations, no evidence of pelvic endometriosis was found [66, 76-82]. Additionally, 58 of 74 cases showed a history of gynecological disorders. These observations support the embolization theory as the underlying cause of ectopic endometriosis in the respiratory tract. While in their case [65] there was no proven pelvic endometriosis or gynecological disease, the patient has previously undergone induced abortions, and there were two cases in the literature review in which induced abortion may have caused endometriosis in the respiratory system [65].

For women in whom pulmonary endometriosis is suspected, a current history of catamenial hemoptysis, active bleeding observed by bronchoscopy, and evidence from CT scans justify the preliminary diagnosis. The endometriosis patient's history, environmental exposures, family history, and physical examination are considered just as important for assessment and care [65]. S P Rachagan et al 1996 [83[, from Malaysia reviewed a rare case of 45 year old woman with pulmonary and umbilical endometriosis who presented as spontaneous pneumothorax in a medical unit. The patient was presenting with right pleuritic chest pain. She gave a two-year history of cyclical haemoptysis and slight bleeding from the umbilicus which occurred during her menses. She also had dysmenorrhoea throughout her menses which lasted for seven days [83].

Pulmonary endometriosis has been described to manifest as either asymptomatic pulmonary nodule or as pneumothorax, haemothorax or cyclical haemoptysis [83]. Karpek et al [84] reviewed in the world literature 84 cases of pulmonary endometriosis, they found that 63 of these cases (75%) presented as catamenial pneumothorax, 9 (10.7%) as catamenial haemothorax, 7 (8.3%) as cyclical haemoptysis and five (6%) as asymptomatic pulmonary nodules. Of these 84 cases with catamenial pneumothorax, 95% occurred in the right chest and 22% had concurrent pelvic endometriosis [83-84].

Fenestration or defects of the diaphragm have been well recognised and are located more commonly in the right diaphragm [83]. A theory has been proposed of a continuous current of peritoneal fluid circulating from the pelvis to the right upper quadrant of the abdomen which if true, would favour the right [70-74, 83]. diaphragmatic area over other areas coming into contact with floating endometriotic particles during retrograde menstruation [83, 85].

Nikolaos Machairiotis et al 2013 [1] mentioned that endometriosis of the thorax is a clinical entity that includes the presence of ectopic endometrial tissue in the pleura, the pericardium and rarely the diaphragm. This is often expressed as catamenial pneumothorax [1]. Catamenial pneumothorax is the most common clinical expression of thoracic endometriosis syndrome, which includes four other entities. These are in brief, catamenial hemothorax, catamenial hemoptysis, endometriotic lung nodules, and catamenial chest pain [1].

For the development of catamenial pneumothorax the presence of endometrial tissue in the thoracic cavity is necessary [1]. There are many theories trying to explain this phenomenon. The theory of Suginamy et al., 1991 [86] suggests that endometrial tissue may circulate along with the peritoneal fluid in the abdominal cavity following a circle "route" down the left peritoneal gutter over the pelvic floor and up the right gutter to the peritoneal surface of the diaphragm. This "route" explains the increased frequency of catamenial pneumothorax of the right side [86] and blebs that may exist in normal lungs [86- 87]. Additionally, to the cases of endometriosis of the lower respiratory system, there are two case reports in the literatures refer to upper respiratory system endometriosis and more specifically to nasal endometriosis [1]. Nasal endometriosis causes cyclic epistaxis and nasal pain, which is synchronous to the menstrual cycle [1, 88]

Endometriosis of Extremities

Most cases of musculoskeletal endometriosis exist without evidence of pelvic disease [89]. The symptoms and signs of disease follow a somewhat predictable course dictated by the anatomic site of involvement. Surgical treatment is most often successful [89].

The case of a patient who had endometriosis in the body of the biceps femoris has been described [91]. Another case of the posterior left thigh has been reported [90], as well as two cases of the right thigh, one anteriorly [92], and one laterally [93]. One case report of endometriosis of the right gluteus maximus exists [94]. The patients ranged in age from 24 to 36 and had noticed progressive pain or localized swelling over the course of months to years [89]. Symptoms were typically worse during menses in most cases. Physical examination would typically show a hard, rubbery, often tender mass, in most cases, although computed tomography (CT) scan was required to diagnose a deeper lesion [94]. Local aggressive surgical excision was curative without the need for postoperative medical therapy in all but one case [89, 92].

A 5cm X 7cm painful soft tissue mass posterior to the right fibular head which appeared over the course of seven months in a 32-year-old black woman was not associated with neuropathy or vascular involvement [89, 95]. The pain and swelling increased during menses. Surgical exploration found the mass extended from the posterior head of the fibula under the lateral head of the gastrocnemius and completely surrounded the peroneal nerve. A biopsy showed endometriosis [89].

A 45-year-old nulliparous woman with right foot drop for six years developed a painful 8cm X 15cm swelling of the right lateral thigh [96]. CT scan showed that this connected through the obturator foramen with a pelvic soft tissue tumor [89].

A 27-year-old nullipara noticed a small slightly painful lump of the left side of her neck which had been growing for about a year [89, 97]. A 2cm ovoid rubbery, mobile mass was removed and microscopy showed endometriosis in the secretory phase. Pelvic and pulmonary examinations were negative [89].

RP Sharma et al 2009 [98], published a case report of a 41-year-old woman with no previous pregnancies or fullterm births presented to the emergency department with swelling of the right lower extremity and pelvic pain. Her symptoms began one week earlier, at which point she was seen by her primary care physician, who diagnosed deep vein thrombosis (DVT) of the right lower extremity. The patient had a medical history significant for infertility, tobacco use and intravenous drug abuse. After diagnostic workup which included a coagulation profile, venous duplex ultrasound of the pelvis and lower extremities, and computed tomography (CT) of the abdomen and pelvis, the diagnosis of endometriosis causing lower extremity deep vein thrombosis was made [98].

Literatures showed two case reports of endometriosis occurring around large veins. The first case reported endometriosis involving the left femoral vein [99]. The patient presented with a painful groin mass that showed characteristics of endometriosis in the adventitial layer of the vein. The second case was due to endometriosis encircling the right external iliac vein causing catamenial edema of the right leg and thigh. Successful surgical resection of the endometriosis was performed [100].The last case is different from the case mentioned in RP Sharma et al [98], Which was no DVT was evident.

Sadegh Saberi et al 2009 [101], presented a case of woman in her late 20s was referred to the orthopedic clinic because of a painful mass in her left leg. Her vague pain had not been accompanied by any systemic symptoms since its onset 2 years earlier. One year after pain onset, sensation of a gradually growing mass began. History of any related trauma was negative. The patient complained that the size of the mass and the intensity of the pain were fluctuating according to her menstrual cycles and were especially exacerbated during her menstrual period. After diagnostic workup the diagnosis of calf endometriosis was made [101].

Endometriosis of the musculoskeletal system has been reported in the pubis, buttocks (gluteus minimus muscle), thigh, knee, shoulder, elbow, forearm, hand, sciatic and obturator nerves, and femoral vein at the saphenous opening [101- 114]. Most cases of extremity endometriosis occur in the groin or anteromedial aspect of the thigh, [101, 110] probably by progression of pelvic endometriosis down the round ligament and into the inguinal canal; however, confirmation of pelvic endometriosis has not consistently been made [115]. In all cases, diagnosis was based on histologic appearance of tissue samples, and patients had local pain as the chief complaint [101].

Central Nervous System Endometriosis:

Although endometriosis is one of the most common human diseases, central nervous system involvement is rare [116]. Sarma et al 2004 [116], described a cystic mass involving the cerebellar vermis, with MRI features of intracystic hemorrhage similar to that described in pelvic endometriomas. Histologic examination was consistent with a diagnosis of endometriosis [116].

Thibodeau et al 1987 [117], described a case of a 20-year-old woman presented with a 3-year history of intermittent focal headaches and a generalized seizure. Computerized tomography demonstrated a hypodense ring-enhancing cystic right parietal lobe lesion. At operation, a chocolate-colored cyst was excised which on histological examination proved to be endometriosis [117].

M. Ichida et al 1993 [118], presented a 31 year patient with cerebral endometriosis. She had repetitive partial seizures on the first day of her menstrual cycle. The seizures were controlled by danazol after the causative lesions were surgically removed [118].

Central nervous system involvement is slightly more frequent in the spine. Cyclical symptoms related to menstruation are often present in patients with central nervous system involvement [116]. One report describes menstruation- related headaches, papilledema, and unresponsiveness caused by cryptogenic subarachnoid hemorrhage from ectopic endometrial tissue in the spine [116, 119].

It hase been found that the cerebellum has features bearing remarkable similarity to MRI appearances of pelvic endometriomas. The shading sign on MRI or any other evidence of hemorrhage in a cystic lesion in a female patient, should alert the radiologist to the possibility of endometriosis even in unusual sites. However, the final diagnosis in such rare locations can, of course, only be made by pathologists [116].

Endometriosis has been described in the spinal cord [89]. Lombardo L et al 1968 [120] described a 26-year-old woman had a five year history of generalized lower extremity muscle and pains with moderate lumbosacral pain radiating to the left leg for two years. Pain increased monthly about five days before menses. Headache, nausea, vomiting, stiffness of the neck and back and a fever caused hospital admission for suspected meningitis. Lumbar puncture showed normal pressure and red blood cells. A myelogram showed a mass at the level of L-1 and L-2. Laminectomy found a round tumor inside the dural sac on the left, measuring up to 1.5cm in diameter. It was adherent to the roots of the cauda equina and two nerve roots were sacrificed for its removal. Photomicrographs illustrating the lesion show clear evidence of endometriosis. The pain was relieved although skin anesthesia in dermatomes L-1 and L-2 on the left side remained. Pain and myelogram evidence of recurrence of the tumor recurred within three months and the patient was treated with progesterone for symptomatic relief [89, 120].

Sun Z et al., 2002 [121], described a case of 27-year-old female patient had progressively worsening lower extremity and lumbar pain for ten years. Weakness and dysuria eventually appeared and the patient eventually could not stand. MRI showed a tumor at the L-4 level of the spinal canal and at surgery the tumor was fused to the cauda equina so that complete removal was impossible. Microscopy confirmed endometriosis [89, 121]. However, Erbayraktar S et al 2002 [122], described a case of 28-year-old woman had a two years history of cyclic low back and groin pain. MRI showed a mass 2.6cm X 1.3cm X 1.4cm in dimension beneath the dura of the lumbar spinal canal. It was incompletely removed. Laparoscopy showed pelvic and intestinal endometriosis and gonadotropin-releasing hormone (GnRH) agonist therapy was administered for 12 months [89,122].

Endometriosis on or near the sciatic nerve is the most common site of involvement of the peripheral nervous system by endometriosis.Approximately 90% of cases are right-sided. Patients may complain of pain in a sciatic distribution occurring just before and during menstruation, sometimes with motor dysfunction of the affected extremity [89, 123-127] The sciatic pain may become chronic in some. Endometriosis usually involves the pelvic portion of the roots of the sciatic nerve without actual invasion of the nerve [89, 123, 128]

As mentioned in above cases scietic nerve is a common site to be involved which is probably because of its anatomical contiguity to the lower pelvis [128-129]. In this instance, clinical manifestation is that of cyclic sciatica, due to compression to the nerve trunks, with characteristic recurrence at menstruation[129]. Characteristic symptomatology was, probably, referable to the presence of endometrioid functional (immunohistochemistry demonstrated expression of oestrogen and progesterone receptors) glands within the mass, causing ectopic extravasations of blood during menstruation, with consequent spinal cord compression [119, 121, 129].

The major clinical characteristics of spinal endometriosis are a series of symptoms associated with the menstrual period with meningeal irritation syndromes, cranial hyper-pressure resulting from recurrent subarachnoid haemorrhage, or symptoms deriving from compression of nidus to nerve tissue of the spinal canal (pain in the lumbar region or lower extremities, dysesthesia of the bladder or rectum, and even paraplegia). There can be also manifestations resulting from local infiltration of nidus, lumbar pain or dyskinesia [129].

Rare Locations of Endometriosis:

Among the other rare locations of endometriosis it is important to refer the endometriosis of large muscles such as the adductor compartment [1, 130], the endometriosis of the rectus abdominis muscle [1, 131].

Ectopic endometrium has been found in the umbilicus, skin, vagina, vulva, cervix, and perineum, in the inguinal canal, upper abdominal peritoneum and organs (liver, spleen), gastrointestinal tract, urinary system, breasts, diaphragm, pleural cavity, brain, eye, lymph nodes, lung and pericardium [7, 132]. Unique cases have also been documented in males [7, 133-134].

References

1. Nikolaos Machairiotis, Aikaterini Stylianaki, Georgios Dryllis, Paul Zarogoulidis, Paraskevi Kouroutou, Nikolaos Tsiamis, et al. Extrapelvic endometriosis: a rare entity or an under diagnosed condition? Diagnostic Pathology 2013; 8:194.

2. Agarwal A, Fong YF. Cutaneous endometriosis. Singapore Med J. 2008; 49:704–9.

3. Blanco RG, Parithivel VS, Shah AK, Gumbs MA, Schein M, Gerst PH. Abdominal wall endometriomas. Am J Surg. 2003; 185:596–8.

4. Pathan SK, Kapila K, Haji BE, Mallik MK, Al-Ansary TA, George SS, et al. Cytomorphological spectrum in scar endometriosis: a study of eight cases. Cytopathology 2005; 16:94–9.

5. Horton JD, Dezee KJ, Ahnfeldt EP, Wagner M. Abdominal wall endometriosis: a surgeon's perspective and review of 445 cases. Am J Surg. 2008;196:207–12.

6. Zaheer Abbas Ali Khan Pathan, US Dinesh, and Ravikala Rao Scar endometriosis J Cytol. 2010 July; 27(3): 106–108.

7. Agarwal N, Subramanian A. Endometriosis - Morphology, clinical presentations and molecular pathology. J Lab Physician 2010;2:1–9.

8. Catalina-Fernández I, López-Presa D, Sáenz-Santamaria J. Fine needle aspiration cytology in cutaneous and subcutaneous endometriosis. Acta Cytol. 2007; 51:380–4.

9. Teh WT, Vollenhoven B, Harris PI. Umbilical endometriosis, a pathology that a gynecologist may encounter when inserting Veres needle. Fertil Steril. 2006; 86(1764):e1–2.

10. Victory R, Diamond MP, Johns DA. Villar's nodule: a case report and systematic literature review of endometriosis externa of the umbilicus. J Minim Invasive Gynecol. 2007; 14:23–32.

11. Chatzikokkinou P, Thorfinn J, Angelidis K I, Papa G, Trevisan G. Spontaneous endometriosis in an umbilical skin lesion. Acta Dermatoven APA. 2008;18:126–30.

12. Saad Suhair Al, Malik Hamdi Mohammed Al-Shinawi, Kumar A, Amallia F. I. Extra-Gonadal Endometriosis: Unusual Presentation. Vol. 29. Medical Bulletin: Bahrain; 2007. Brair. Extra-Gonadal Endometriosis: Unusual Presentation; pp. 1–11.

13. Razzi S, Rubegni P, Sartini A, De Simone S, Fava A, Cobellis L, et al. Umbilical endometriosis in pregnancy: a case report. Gynecol Endocrinol. 2004; 18:114–6.

14. Michael K. Elm, James V. Twede, George W. Turiansky. Primary cutaneous endometriosis of the umbilicus: A case report. Cutis. 2008; 81:124-126.

15. Hussain M, Noorani K. Primary umbilical endometriosis— a rare variant of cutaneous endometriosis. J Coll Physicians Surg Pak. 2003;13:164-165.

16. Okunlola MA, Adekunle AO, Arowojolu AO, et al. Isolated umbilical endometriosis—a rare finding. Afr J Med Med Sci. 2002; 31:281-282.

17. von Stemm AMR, Meigel WN, Scheidel P, et al. Umbilical endometriosis. J Eur Acad Dermatol Venereol. 1999;12:30-32.

18. Zollner U, Girschick G, Steck T, et al. Umbilical endometriosis without previous pelvic surgery: a case report. Arch Gynecol Obstet. 2003;267:258-260.

19. Scholefield HJ, Sajjad Y, Morgan PR. Cutaneous endometriosis and its association with caesarean section and gynaecological procedures. J Obstet Gynaecol. 2002;22:553-554.

20. Friedman PM, Rico MJ. Cutaneous endometriosis. Dermatol Online J. 2000;6:8.

21. Antonelli A, Simeone C, Frego E, et al. Surgical treatment of ureteral obstruction from endometriosis: our experience with thirteen cases. Int Urogynecol J Pelvic Floor Dysfunct. 2004; 15:407–12.

22. Ball TL, Platt MA. Urologic complications of endometriosis. Am J Obstet Gynecol. 1962;84:1516–21.

23. Denes FT, Pompeo ACL, Momtellato NID. Ureteral endometriosis. Int Urol Nephrol. 1980;12:205–9.

24. Dick AL, Lang DW, Bergman RT. Postmenopausal endometriosis with ureteral obstruction. Br J Urol. 1973;45:153 5.

25. Stanley KE, Utz DC, Dockerty MB. Clinically significant endometriosis of the urinary tract. Surg Gynecol Obstet. 1965;120:491–5.

26. Stillwell TJ, Kramer SA, Lee RA. Endometriosis of ureter. Urology. 1986;28:81–5.

27. Jubanyik KJ, Comite F. Extrapelvic endometriosis. Obstet Gynecol Clin North Am. 1997; 24:411–40.

28. Andrew Feifer, Mona Ala El-Din, Atilla Omeroglu, and Maurice Anidjar. Obstructive uropathy associated with primary ureteral

endometrioma: case report and review of the literature Can Urol Assoc J. 2009; 3(3): E10–E130.

29. Maccagnano C, Freschi M, Ghezzi M, Rocchini L, Pellucchi F, Rigatti P, Montorsi F, Colombo R: Kidney endometriosis. Minerva urologica enefrologica 2013, 65:157–159.

30. Gupta K, Rajwanshi A, Srinivasan R: Endometriosis of the kidney: diagnosis by fine-needle aspiration cytology. Diagn Cytopathol 2005, 33:60–61.

31. Papakonstantinou E, Orfanos F, Mariolis-Sapsakos T, Vlahodimitropoulos D, Kondi-Pafiti A: A rare case of intrinsic ureteral endometriosis causing hydronephrosis in a 40-year-old woman. A case report and literature review. Clin Exp Obstet Gynecol 2012, 39:265–268.

32. Horn LC, Do Minh M, Stolzenburg JU: Intrinsic form of ureteral endometriosis causing ureteral obstruction and partial loss of kidney function. Urol Int 2004, 73:181–184.

33. Antonelli A: Urinary tract endometriosis. Urologia 2012, 79:167–170.

34. Aliasghar Yarmohamadi and Nasser Mogharabian (2012). Urinary Tract Endometriosis, Endometriosis – Basic Concepts and Current Research Trends, Prof. Koel Chaudhury (Ed.), ISBN: 978-953-51-0524-4, InTech, Available from:

http://www.intechopen.com/books/endometriosis-basic-concepts-and-current-researchtrends/ urinary-tract-endometriosis. Accessed 22th March 2014.

35. Clement PB. Springer-Verlag: New York; 1994. Blaustein's pathology of the female genital tract; pp. 660–80.

36. Gedgaudas-McClees RK. Philadelphia: Saunders; 1994. Gastrointestinal complications of gynecologic diseases In: Textbook of gastrointestinal radiology; pp. 2559–67.

37. Zwas FR, Lyon DT. Endometriosis.An important condition in clinical gastroenterology. Dig Dis Sci. 1991;36:353–64.

38. Goldsmith PJ, Ahmad N, Dasgupta D, Campbell J, Guthrie JA, Lodge JP. Case hepatic endometriosis: a continuing diagnostic dilemma. HPB Surg. 2009; 407206.

39. Heejin Lee Kyu-Rae Kim. Intestinal Endometriosis: Clinicopathologic Analysis of 15 Cases Including a Case of Endometrioid Adenocarcinoma. The Korean Jrnl of Patho. 2009;43:120–5.

40. Al Oulaqi NS, Hefny AF, Joshi S, Salim K, Abu-Zidan FM. Endometriosis of the appendix. Afr Health Sci. 2008; 8:196–8.

41. Gustofson RL, Kim N, Liu S, Stratton P. Endometriosis and the

appendix: a case series and comprehensive review of the literature. Fertil Steril. 2006;86:298–303.

42. Yantiss RK, Clement PB, Young RH. Endometriosis of the intestinal tract: a study of 44 cases of a disease that may cause diverse challenges in clinical and pathologic evaluation. Am J Surg Pathol. 2001;25:445–54.

43. Driman DK, Melega DE, Vilos GA, Plewes EA. Mucocele of the appendix secondary to endometriosis.Report of two cases, one with localized pseudomyxoma peritonei. Am J Clin Pathol. 2000;113:860–4.

44. Bailey HR, Ott MT, Hartendorp P: Aggressive surgical management for advanced colorectal endometriosis. Dis Colon Rectum 1994, 37:747–753.

45. Gustofson RL, Kim N, Liu S, Stratton P: Endometriosis and the appendix: a case series and comprehensive review of the literature. Fertil Steril 2006, 86:298–303.

46. Jatan AK, Solomon MJ, Young J, Cooper M, Pathma-Nathan N: Laparoscopic management of rectal endometriosis. Dis Colon Rectum 2006, 49:169–174.

47. Maroun P, Cooper MJ, Reid GD, Keirse MJ: Relevance of gastrointestinal symptoms in endometriosis. Aust N Z J Obstet Gynaecol 2009, 49:411–414.

48. Jerby BL, Kessler H, Falcone T, Milsom JW: Laparoscopic management of colorectal endometriosis. Surg Endosc 1999, 13:1125–1128.

49. Goldsmith PJ, Ahmad N, Dasgupta D, Campbell J, Guthrie JA, Lodge JP: Case hepatic endometriosis: a continuing diagnostic dilemma. HPB Surg 2009, 2009:407206.

50. Bouras AF, Vincentelli A, Boleslawski E, Truant S, Liddo G, Prat A, Pruvot FR, Zerbib P: Liver endometriosis presenting as a liver mass associated with high blood levels of tumoral biomarkers. Clin Res Hepatol Gastroenterol 2013, 37:e85–88.

51. Fluegen G, Jankowiak F, Zacarias Foehrding L, Kroepil F, Knoefel WT, Topp SA: Intrahepatic endometriosis as differential diagnosis: case report and literature review. WJG 2013, 19:4818–4822.

52. Kalkur S, Raza A, Richardson RE: Right upper quadrant pain? Think outside the liver: A case of diaphragmatic perihepatic endometriosis. J Obstet Gynaecol 2013, 33:743.

53. Watari H, Shibahara N, Ebisawa S, Nogami T, Fujimoto M, Hikiami H, Shimada Y: [Case report; A case of hepatic endometriosis with periodic right upper quadrant pain]. Nihon Naika Gakkai zasshi 2012,

101:3233–3235.

54. Saldana DG, de Acosta DA, Aleman HP, Gebrehiwot D, Torres E: Gallbladder endometrioma associated with obstructive jaundice and a serous ovarian cystic adenoma. South Med J 2010, 103:1250–1252.

55. Lia C. Kaufman, Thomas C. Smyrk, Michael J. Levy, Felicity T. Enders, and Amy S. Oxentenko. Symptomatic Intestinal Endometriosis Requiring Surgical Resection: Clinical Presentation and Preoperative Diagnosis Am J Gastroenterol 2011; 106:1325– 1332.

56. Yu-Hung Lin, Li-Jen Kuo, Ai-Ying Chuang, Tsun-I Cheng, Chi-Feng Hung. Extrapelvic endometriosis complicated with colonic obstruction. J Chin Med Assoc 2006; 69 (1): 47-50.

57. Cameron IC, Rogers S, Collins MC, Reed MWR. Intestinal endometriosis: presentation, investigation, and surgical management. Int J Colorectal Dis 1995;10:83–6.

58. Stratton P, Winkel C, Premkumar A, Chow C, Wilson J, Hearns-Strokes R, Heo S, et al. Diagnostic accuracy of laparoscopy, magnetic resonance imaging, and histopathologic examination for the detection of endometriosis. Fertil Steril 2003;79:1078–85.

59. Meyers WC, Kelvin FM, Jones RS. Diagnosis and surgical treatment

of colonic endometriosis. Arch Surg 1979;114: 169–75.

60. Duepree HJ, Senagore AJ, Delaney CP, Marcello PW, Brady KM, Falcone T. Laparoscopic resection of deep pelvic endometriosis with rectosigmoid involvement. J Am Coll Surg 2002;195:754–8.

61. Suhair Al- Saad, Hamdi Mohammed Al-Shinawi, Malik Ashok Kumar, Amallia F.I.Brair. Extra-Gonadal Endometriosis: Unusual Presentation. Bahrain Medical Bulletin 2007; 29(1): 1-11.

62. Gustofson R L, Kim N, Liu S. Endometriosis and the appendix: a case series and comprehensive review of the literature. Fertil Steril. 2006,86: 298-303.

63. Tade AO. Chronic intestinal obstruction due to rectosigmoid endometriosis: a case report. Niger J. Med. 2006;15: 165-6.

64. Paksoy M, Karabicak I, Avan F. Intestinal obstruction due to rectal endometriosis. Mt Sinai J Med. 2005;72: 405-8.

65. Haidong Huang, Chen Li, Paul Zarogoulidis, Kaid Darwiche, Nikolaos Machairiotis, Lixin Yang, et al. Endometriosis of the lung: report of a case and literature review. European Journal of Medical Research 2013;18:13.

66. Giudice LC, Kao LC: Endometriosis. Lancet 2004, 364(9447):1789–1799.

67. Suginami H, Hamada K, Yano K: A case of endometriosis of the lung treated with danazol. Obstet Gynecol 1985, 66(3 Suppl):68S–71S.

68. Park YB, Heo GM, Moon HK, Cho SJ, Shin YC, Eom KS, Kim CH, Lee JY, Mo EK, Jung KS: Pulmonary endometriosis resected by video-assisted thoracoscopic surgery. Respirology 2006, 11(2):221–223.

69. Shiota Y, Umemura S, Arikita H, Horita N, Hiyama J, Tetsuya Ono T, Sasaki N, Taniyama K, Yamakido M: A case of parenchymal pulmonary endometriosis, diagnosed by cytologic examination of bronchial washing. Respiration 2001, 68(4):439.

70. Joseph J, Reed CE, Sahn SA. Thoracic endometriosis. Recurrence following hysterectomy with bilateral salpingo-oophorectomy and successful treatment with talc pleurodesis. Chest. 1994;106:1894–96.

71. Lee CY, Di Loreto PC, Beaudoin J. Catamenial pneumothorax. Obstet Gynecol. 1974;44:407–11.

72. Crosby DJ. Catamenial pneumothorax. Ariz Med. 1973;30:260–61.

73. Hibbard LT, Schumann WR, Goldstein GE. Thoracic endometriosis: a review and report of two cases. Am J Obstet Gynecol. 1981;140:227–32.

74. Yusuf N, Haque M A, Rahman M H, Ali M A. An Atypical

Presentation of A Case of Endometriosis. TAJ. 2006;19:27–30.

75. Agrawal A, Nation J, Ghatage P, Chu P, Ross S, Magliocco A. Malignant chest wall endometriosis: a case report and literature review. J Obstet Gynaecol Can. 2009;31:538–41.

76. Lattes R, Shepard F, Tovell H, Wylie R: A clinical and pathologic study of endometriosis of the lung. Surg Gynecol Obstet 1956, 103(5):552–558.

77. Fleishman SJ, Davidson JF: Vicarious menstruation, a likely case of pulmonary endometriosis. Lancet 1959, 2(7093):88–89.

78. Granberg I, Willems JS: Endometriosis of lung and pleura diagnosed by aspiration biopsy. Acta Cytol 1977, 21(2):295–297.

79. Suginami H, Hamada K, Yano K: A case of endometriosis of the lung treated with danazol. Obstet Gynecol 1985, 66(3 Suppl):68S–71S.

80. Muller A, Dubach UC: Extragenital endometriosis. Report of a case of pulmonary endometriosis. Schweiz Med Wochenschr 1971, 101(34):1247– 1250.

81. Taccagni GL, Beretta E, Radice F, Staudacher C, Sironi M: Pulmonary endometriosis: presentation of a case and review of the

literature. Pathologica 1985, 77(1051):539–548.

82. Castillo A, Meneses M, Rosa G, Saldias F: Pulmonary endometriosis. Clinical case. Rev Med Chil 1991, 119(6):683–686.

83. S P Rachagan, S Zawiah, A Menon. Extra pelvic endometriosis and catamenial pneumothorax. Med J Malaysia 1996; 51(4): 480-481.

84. Karpek JP, Appel D, Merav A : Pulmonary endometriosis. Lung 1985;163 : 151.

85. Foster DC, Stern JL, Buscema J et al. Pleura! and parenchyma! pulmonary endometriosis. Ob stet Gynecol 1981;58 : 552.

86. Suginami H: A reappraisal of the coelomic metaplasia theory by reviewing endometriosis occurring in unusual sites and instances. Am J Obstet Gynecol 1991, 165:214–218.

87. Korom S, Canyurt H, Missbach A, Schneiter D, Kurrer MO, Haller U, Keller PJ, Furrer M, Weder W: Catamenial pneumothorax revisited: clinical approach and systematic review of the literature. J Thorac Cardiovasc Surg 2004, 128:502–508.

88. Mignemi G, Facchini C, Raimondo D, Montanari G, Ferrini G, Seracchioli R: A case report of nasal endometriosis in a patient affected by Behcet's disease. J Minim Invasive Gynecol 2012, 19:514–516.

89. David B. Redwine. Musculoskeletal endometriosis. Available in

http://endopaedia.info/index.html. Accessed 23th March 2014.

90. Giangarra C, Gallo G, Newman R, Dorfman H. Endometriosis in the biceps femoris. J Bone Joint Surg 1987;69:290-2.

91. Schlicke CP. Ectopic endometrial tissue in the thigh. JAMA 1946;132:445-6.

92. Gitelis S, Petasnick JP, Turner DA, Ghiselli RW, Miller III AW. Endometriosis simulating a soft tissue tumor of the thigh: CT and MR evaluation. J Comput Assist Tomogr 1985;9: 573-6.

93. Nunn LL. Endometrioma of the thigh. North-west Med 1949;48:474-5.

94. Butha AJ, Halliday AEG, Flanagan JP. Endometriosis in gluteus muscle with surgical implantation. A case report. Act Orthop Scan 1991;62:497-9.

95. Patel VC, Samuels H, Abeles E, Hirjibiehedin PF. Endometriosis at the knee. A case report. Clin Orthop Rel Res 1982;171:140-4.

96. Oei SG, Peters AAW, Welvaart K, Bode PJ, Fleuren G-J. Aggressive endometriosis in bone. Lancet 1992;339:1477-8 (Letter).

97. Gennari L, Luciani L. Un caso di endometriosi del muscolo trapezio. Tumori 1964;51:361-5.

98. RP Sharma, F Delly, H Marin, S Sturza. Endometriosis causing

lower extremity deep vein thrombosis – case report and review of the literature. Int J Angiol 2009; 18(4):199-202.

99. Recalde AL, Majmudar B. Endometriosis involving the femoral vein. South Med J 1977; 70:69-74.

100. Rosengarten AM, Wong J, Gibbons S. Endometriosis causing cyclic compression of the right external iliac vein with cyclic edema of the right leg and thigh. J Obstet Gynaecol Can 2002;24:33-5.

101. Sadegh Saberi, Amir Reza Farhoud, and Ali Radmehr. Calf Endometriosis: A Case report and review of musculoskeletal involvement. Am J Orthop 2009;38(11):E175-E178.

102. Botha AJ, Halliday AE, Flanagan JP. Endometriosis in gluteus muscle with surgical implantation. A case report. Acta Orthop Scand. 1991; 62(5):497- 499.

103. Das Gupta S, Pal SK, Saha PK, Dawn CS. Endometriosis in the thumb. *J* Indian Med Assoc. 1985;83(4):122-123.

104. Duncan C, Pitney WR. Endometrial tumors in the extremities. *Med J Aust.* 1949;2(20):715-717.

105. Strasser EJ, Davis RM. Extraperitoneal inguinal endometriosis. Am J Surg. 1977;43(6):421-422.

106. Patel VC, Samuels H, Abeles E, Hirjibehedin PF. Endometriosis at

the knee. Clin Orthop. 1982;(171):140-144.

107. Aron SE. Endometriosis in the region of the deltoid muscle [in Russian]. Arkh Patol. 1957;19(7):67-68.

108. Basu PA, Kesani AK, Stacy GS, Peabody TD. Endometriosis of the vastus lateralis muscle. Skeletal Radiol. 2006;35(8):595-598.

109. Pellegrini VD Jr, Pasternak HS, Macaulay WP. Endometrioma of the pubis: a differential in the diagnosis of hip pain. A report of two cases. J Bone Joint Surg Am. 1981;63(8):1333-1334.

110. Recalde AL, Majmudar B. Endometriosis involving the femoral vein. South Med J. 1977;70(1):69-74.

111. Baker GS, Parsons WR, Welch JS. Endometriosis in the sheath of the sciatic nerve. J Neurosurg. 1966;25(6):652-655.

112. Forrest J, Brooks DL. Cyclic sciatica of endometriosis. JAMA. 1972; 222(9):1177-1178.

113. Hibbard J, Schreiber J. Footdrop due to a sciatic nerve endometriosis. Am J Obstet Gynecol. 1984;149(7):800-801.

114. Redwine DB, Sharpe DR. Endometriosis of the obturator nerve. A case report. J Reprod Med. 1990;35(4):434-435.

115. Ball TL, Platt MA. Urologic complications of endometriosis. Am J Obstet Gynecol. 1962;84:1516-1521.

116. Sarma D, Iyengar P, Marotta TR, terBrugge KG, Gentili F, Halliday W. Cerebellar endometriosis. AJR Am J Roentgenol. 2004;182:1543-6.

117. Thibodeau LL, Prioleau GR, Manuelidis EE, Merino MJ, Heafner MD. Cerebral endometriosis.Case report. J Neurosurg. 1987;66:609-10.

118. M. Ichida, A. Gomi, N. Hiranouchi, K. Fujimoto, K. Suzuki, M. Yoshida, M. Nokubi, T. Masuzawa.. A case of cerebral endometriosis causing catamenial epilepsy *Neurology* 1993; 43(12): 2708-09

119. Duke R, Fawcett P, Booth J. Recurrent subarachnoid hemorrhage due to endometriosis. Neurology 1995;45:1000-1002

120. . Lombardo L, Mateos JH, Barroeta FF. Subarachnoid hemorrhage due to endometriosis of the spinal canal. Neurology 1968;18:423-6.

121. Sun Z, Wang Y, Zhao L, Ma L. Intraspinal endometriosis: A case report. Chin Med J 2002; 115:622-3.

122. Erbayraktar S, Acar B, Saygili U, Kargi A, Acar U. Management of intramedullary endometriosis of the conus medullaris. A case report. J Reprod Med 2002;47:955-8.

123. Denton RO, Sherrill JD. Sciatic syndrome due to endometriosis of sciatic nerve. South Med J 1955;48:1027-31.

124. Hibbard J, Schreiber JR. Footdrop due to sciatic nerve

endometriosis. Am J Obstet Gynecol 1984; 149:800-1.

125. Salazar-Grueso E, Roos R. Sciatic endometriosis: A treatable sensorimotor mononeuropathy. Neurology 1986;36:1360-3.

126. Torkelson SJ, Lee RA, Hildahl DB. Endometriosis of the sciatic nerve: A report of two cases and a review of the literature. Obstet Gynecol 1988; 71:473-7.

127. Liberman JS, Trelford J, Taylor R, Garrett V. Neurological deficits, back pain tied to endometriosis. JAMA 1983;249:686.

128. Baker GS, Parsons WR, Welch JS. Endometriosis within the sheath of the sciatic nerve. J Neurosurg 1966;25:652-5.

129. V. Barresi, S. Cerasoli, E. Vitarelli and R. Donati. Spinal intradural müllerianosis: a case report. Histol Histopathol 2006; 21: 1111-1114

130. Fambrini M, Andersson KL, Campanacci DA, Vanzi E, Bruni V, Buccoliero AM, Pieralli A, Livi L, Scarselli G: Large-muscle endometriosis involving the adductor tight compartment: case report. J Minim Invasive Gynecol 2010, 17:258–261.

131. Kandil E, Alabbas H, Ghafar M, Burris K, Sawas A, Schwartzman A: Endometriosis in the rectus abdominis muscle: case report and literature review. J La State Med Soc 2009, 161:321–324.

132. Sensenig DM, Serlin O, Hawthorne HR. Pericardial endometriosis.

An experimental study in dogs. JAMA 1966; 198: 645-7.

133. Martin JD Jr, Haucl AE. Endometriosis in the male. Am Surg 1985; 51: 426-30.

134. Schrodt Gr, Alcorn MO, Ibanez J. Endometriosis of the male urinary system. J Urol 1980; 124: 722-3.

6 CATAMENIAL ENDOMETRIOSIS

Even at the cost of repetition we have touched upon this subject because the condition is being increasingly recognised and it is of paramount importance to be aware of this menacing condition. Notwithstanding catamenial endometriosis has been known for several decades, it has not received hitherto the attention it deserves and was relegated to the status of an extremely rare condition. The condition has now become increasingly recognized and several studies have appeared in the literature [1].

Recent reports signify that its incidence may be more common than historically believed [2-4]. Prior to the dawn of video-assisted thoracoscopy in 1990, surgical management of recurrent spontaneous pneumothorax was axillary thoracotomy and apical pleurectomy, which did not always permit proper examination of the diaphragm [5]. The diagnosis of catamenial pneumothorax may have thus been missed, possibly accounting for its low incidence pre-1990 [6].

Catamenial pneumothorax accounts for about a third of cases of spontaneous pneumothoraces in women referred for surgery [7]. It is encountered in 3-6% of spontaneous pneumothorax cases among menstruating women. The percentage among women referred for surgery is significantly higher (25-30%) [8].

Epidemiology:

Unlike the earlier reports of incidence of catamenial pneumothorax which was about 3-6% recent reports of appraisal emerging from studies including larger cohort of patients is that it occurs in 25-30% of primary spontaneous pneumothoraces in females [9-12]. Video assisted thoracoscopic surgery (VATS) has helped considerably to enhanced recognition and diagnosis [11]. This , however , does not embrace the secondary spontaneous pneumothorax secondary to other pulmomary diseases and noncatamenial primary spontaneous pneumothorax [9], while it is predomonatly right sided , it may affect left side or both sides [9-10, 13].

Pneumothorax gnerally affects older age group compared to pelvic endometriosis. The mean age of those effected are in their 3rd or 4th decade of life with age range of 19-45 [9, 13-14]. The average number of attacks before recognition and definitive treatment is 3-5. No genetic or familial patterns have been ascribed to this entity [14].

Thoracic endometriosis syndroem (TES) comprises principally four clinical entities: catamenial pneumothorax (CP), catamenial hemothorax (CHt), catamenial hemoptysis (CH), and lung nodules., CP among them,is the most frequent clinical presentation [15].

CP, CHt, CH, and lung nodules encompass the main clinical entities in TES, but they are not the exclusive manifestations of TES. The sole presentation of TES may be a catamenial pain-only syndrome,to wit cyclic shoulder, neck, epigastric, or right upper quadrant pain,linked with diaphragmatic-only endometriosis cases, explicitly [16-17].

Pathogenesis:

No universally accepted explanation is available for the pathogenesis of the pneumothorax [18]. However , as usual,,numerous pathogenic mechanisms have been postulated [19-22]. Findings of surgical explorations substatntiate the theory of transabdominal-transdiaphragmaticpassage of air to elucidate the pathogenesis of catamenial pneumothorax [23]. These comprise sloughing of pleural implants with consequent air leak, spontaneous rupture of blebs during hormonal changes or peripheral alveolar rupture resultant from the bronchiolar spasm due to prostaglandin secretion of lung endometrial implants and movement of air through the uterus and fallopian tubes into the abdomen and through diaphragmatic opening into the thorax. An absent cervical mucous plug may result in air tracking from the genital tract into the peritoneum and via diaphragmatic fenestrations into the pleural space [22]. In most cases it is related to thoracic endometriosis and/or diaphragmatic fenestrations [24].

According to the hormonal theory, vasospasm due to elevated prostaglandin F_2 at ovulation, may lead to pulmonary ischemia. This, consecutively coupled with prostaglandin-induced bronchospasm, may cause alveolar rupture and subsequent pneumothorax [25]. Synchronous elevations of prostaglandin F2 during menstruation could provoke CPT [26]. When the prostaglandins reach the top levels during sloughing of the endometrial mucosa, the intense constrictor effect of prostaglandin F2 may burst preformed subpleural blebs.. Blebs or bullae may also be more liable to rupture during hormonal changes [27-29]. This hypothesis could account for some explored cases of , bullae or blebs were the only lesions discovered [30].

According to the migration theory, endometrial diaphragmatic implants may come from movement of endometrial tissue from uterus to pelvis, and via the peritoneal flow to the subdiaphragmatic area (specially the right, through the right paracolic gutter, due to clockwise peritoneal circulation, and the "piston" action of the liver). Cyclical necrosis of diaphragmatic endometrial implants can result in diaphragmatic defect(s). Endometrial tissue has been observed on the edges of such defects in many cases of CP. Endometrial cells can pass through the created diaphragmatic defect(s) and spread into the thoracic cavity, including the visceral pleura. Cyclical necrosis, or sloughing and apoptosis of the visceral pleura endometrial implants may lead to rupture of the underlying alveolus and pneumothorax [27-28].

As for the metastatic or lymphovascular microembolization theory: metastatic disssemination spread (or microembolization) of endometrial cells to the lungs via the venous system or the transdiaphragmatic lymphatics, and cyclical necrosis of pulmonary parenchymal foci close to the pleura may cause air leaks. Centrally located lesions may cause haemoptysis [27, 31].

Signs and Symptoms

CP by definfition is recurrent pneumothorax occurring within 72 hours from the start of menstruation [32]. Typically, although it occurs in women aged 30–40 years, it has been diagnosed in young girls at 10 years of age and in post menopausal women most with a history of pelvic endometriosis. CP is the most common manifestation of TES, accounting to nearly 80% of cases. Less common clinical entities include CHt (14%), CH (5%), and lung nodules [33-34]. CP is characteristically cyclic,.The typical clinical manifestations of catamenial pneumothorax comprise spontaneous pneumothorax during or preceding menses, pain, dyspnoea and cough. Thoracic pain before or during menstruation, history of previous spontaneous pneumothorax, symptoms of pelvic endometriosis, history of primary or secondary infertility, with or without diagnosis of previous pelvic endometriosis, history of previous gynaecologic procedure [35-41], and seldom history of catamenial haemoptysis [38,42], may be present Although Catamenial Pneumothrax is generally mild to moderate, they can infrequently be life-threatening [42].

Majority of cases of CP show right sided involvement. Patients with CP manifest symptoms of spontaneous pneumothorax that are usually nonspecific, such as pleurisy, cough, and dyspnoea.. Patients may suffer from peri-scapular or radiating neck pain secondary to diaphragmatic irritation. While most of cases have mild to moderate symptoms it is rare to encounter severe presentations [43].

CHt is an uncommon manifestation of TES [44]. It is similar to CP, both in ts prsentation as well as site of involvement. They may be associated with varaible hemorrhagic effusion.. Both CH and lung nodules constitute clinical entities of bronchopulmonary TES and are extremely rare. Hemoptysis is quite capricious and is neither heavy nor fatal ..It may not always be associated with menstruation. CH and lung nodules being reciprocally related , patients who manifest with CH frequently have lung nodules on imaging studies and vice versa [43].

CP, CHt, CH, and lung nodules symbolize the chief clinical entities in TES. But , they are not the sole manifestations of TES. Explicvitly in the diaphragmatic-only endometriosis cases, catamenial phrenic nerve irritation inducing a catamenial pain-only syndrome, namely cyclic shoulder, neck, epigastric, or right upper quadrant pain, may be the only presentation of TES [45-46].

Overall, a high level of clinical suspicion is of paramount importance in TES. A detailed history might make the difference in promptly establishing a correct diagnosis and avoiding delays in treatment, which are commonly reported.

Diagnosis:

The diagnosis of catamenial pneumothorax can be covertly suggested by excessive recurrences of pneumothorax in a woman of reproductive age with endometriosis. CA-125 is elevated..The diagnosis of catamenial pneumothorax should be considered when a women aged between 30 and 40 years presents with complaints of recurrent right-sided chest pain temporally associated with menstruation [47].

Video-assisted thoracoscopy is useful for confirmation .VATS is the gold standard for the definitive diagnosis as well as surgical treatment of CP [48-50].

Video-assisted thoracic surgery has revealed , diaphragmatic defects and nodules as the most common findings. Pathology establishes endometriosis in most cases.. Endometrialimplants in visceral pleura are also found, albeit less often. Findings ofsurgical explorations favour the hypohesis of transabdominal-transdiaphragmatic migration of air to account for the pathogenesis of catamenial pneumothorax [51].

There must be a high level of suspicion which will be beneficial in the diagnosis of thoracic endometriosis is a high level of clinical suspicion [52].

A cyclic constellation of symptoms can be regarded characteristic of the disease.Nevertheless there is often a delay for more than 8 months from the start of symptoms [53].

Chest X'rays , CT, magnetic resonance imaging, thoracocentesis, and bronchoscopy are not only useful in the diagnosis of the patient manifesting pneumothorax, hemothorax, hemoptysis, or lung nodules but also help exclude malignancy, infection, and other pathologies [54]. However,all these aids provide limited diagnostic value in the diagnosis of TES per se, with variable and inconsistent findings [55-56].

The disadvantage is that in the case of bronchopulmonary endometriosis, bronchoscopy-directed biopsies of suspected lesions generally fail to offer a tissue diagnosis;on the otherhand brush cytology often displays pathognomonic features of endometrial cells [57].

Cytologic smears exhibit characteristic sheets ofepithelial cells and fragments of loosely arranged spindled stroma. It may also show hemosiderin-laden macrophages [58].

An alterntaive appraoch is a combined VATS and laparoscopy procedure in a single session . This approach to treat TES emphasised the need for inspecting the abdominal side of the diaphragm for complete treatment of TES [59]

It may be especially crucial in cases of inconclusive VATS, which may be due to the existence of endometriosis only in the abdominal part of the diaphragm responsible for catamenial phrenic nerve irritation and pain [60].

Pathology:

Grossly, these lesions look red, purple, violet, blueberry, brown, white, gray, or even black in color. Usually they are found on the diaphragmatic central tendon. White nodules indicate healing by fibrosis. The endometrial implants represent normal endometrial tissues in the thorax. They consist of stroma and glands in different stages and present in a wide variety of different shapes and sizes [61-62]. They are lined by pseudo stratified cuboidal epithelium. The glands are of the proliferative type demonste inconspicuous nucleoli, scant eosinophilic cytoplasm, and frequent mitosis. The stroma cells demonstrate limited cytoplasm, mixed extravasated erythrocytes and hemosiderin-laden macrophages [63]. The secretory phase features are not seen. They form cysts with different colors on gross examination as mentioned earlier and sometimes the name "chocolate cyst" is given. Hemorrhage, fibrosis, and inflammatory cell infiltration can be seen in association with these features. The endometrial stroma can be found in the lung parenchyma, within the broncho-vascular bundles or outside the alveolar septa. On immunohistochemistry (IHC) examination, the glands stain positively to many cytokeratins including cytokeratin-7, BER-EP4, and nuclear staining for progesterone and estrogen. The stroma stains positively for vimetin frequently and sometimes for desmin, actin, as well as progesterone and estrogen. None have shown any reaction to epithelial or neuroendocrine stains [64]. Pulmonary hemorrhage and hemosiderin containing macrophages indicates a nearby endometriosis [64-65]

Treatment

Surgery is the treatment of choice in the management of patients with catamenial pneumothorax. If feasible by video-assisted technology,will be advantageous to collect samples for histologic confirmation of endometriosis and to treat the main pathogenic mechanisms ofpneumothorax. Partial diaphragmatic resection and/or exeresis of visceral pleuralimplants, as well as talc pleurodesis, are currently frequently performed . Given the systemic nature of the disease, surgical intervention should, in all cases, be followed by gonadotrophin-releasing hormone (GnRH) analogue therapy to reduce the rate of recurrence [66].

Medical therapy to achieve ovarian rest is imperative in the postoperative period, the multimodality management is the key to ensure success of treatment in this condition [51].

References

1. Guang-Qiong Hou, Bee-Song Chang, Senzan Hsu, Sheng-Po Kao, Dah-Ching Ding. Catamenial Pneumothorax due to Pulmonary Endometriosis- A Case Report. Tzu Chi Med J 2006; 18:305-307.

2. Korom S, Canyurt H, Missbach A. Catamenial pneumothorax revisited: clinical approach and systematic review of the literature. J Thorac Cardiovasc Surg. 2004; 128:502–8.

3. Alifano M, Roth T, Broet S, Schussler O, Magdeleinat P, Regnard J. Catamenial pneumothorax: a prospective study. Chest. 2003;124:1004–8.

4. Marshall M, Ahmed Z, Kucharczuk J. Catamenial pneumothorax: optimal hormonal and surgical management. Eur J Cardiothorac Surg. 2005;27:662–6.

5. Deslauriers J, Beaulieu M, Despres J, Lemieux M, Leblanc J, Desmeules M. Transaxillary pleurectomy for treatment of spontaneous pneumothorax. Ann Thorac Surg 1980;30:569–74.

6. Annabelle C Leong, Aman S Coonar, and Loïc Lang- Lazdunski Catamenial Pneumothorax: Surgical Repair of the Diaphragm and Hormone Treatment Ann R Coll Surg Engl 2006; 88(6): 547–549).

7. Alifano M. Catamenial pneumothorax. Curr Opin Pulm Med. 2010; 16(4):381-6.

8. Visouli AN, Darwiche K, Mpakas A, Zarogoulidis P, Papagiannis A, Tsakiridis K, Machairiotis N, Stylianaki A, Katsikogiannis N, Courcoutsakis N, Zarogoulidis K. Catamenial pneumothorax: a rare entity? Report of 5 cases and review of the literature. J Thorac Dis. 2012;4(Suppl 1):17-31.

9. Visouli AN, Darwiche K, Mpakas A, Zarogoulidis P, Papagiannis A, Tsakiridis K, et al. Catamenial pneumothorax: a rare entity? Report of 5 cases and review of the literature. J Thorac Dis 2012; 4 Suppl 1: S17-S31.

10. Rafay M, El-Bawab H, Kurdli W, Al Kattan K. Diaphragmatic fenestrations in catamenial pneumothorax: a management strategy. Asian Cardiovasc Thorac Ann 2009; 17: 70-72.

11. Yasui S, Taniguchi Y, Suzuki Y, Makihara K, Okada K, Ito N, et al. A Case of Catamenial Pneumothorax Treated by Video- Assisted Thoracoscopic Surgery. Yonago Acta Medica 2003; 46: 25-28.

12. Leong AC, Coonar AS, Lang-Lazdunski L. Catamenial

pneumothorax: surgical repair of the diaphragm and hormonal treatment. Ann R Coll Surg Engl 2006; 88: 547-549.

13. Laws HL, Fox LS, Younger JB. Bilateral catamenial pneumothorax. Arch Surg 1977; 112: 627-628.

14. Tsunezuka Y, Sato H, Kodama T, Shimizu H, Kurumaya H. Expression of CA125 in thoracic endometriosis in a patient with catamenial pneumothorax. Respiration 1999; 66: 470-472.

15. Joseph J, Sahn SA. Thoracic endometriosis syndrome: new observations from an analysis of 110 cases. Am J Med. Feb 1996;100(2):164.

16. Nezhat C, Seidman DS, Nezhat F. Laparoscopic surgical management of diaphragmatic endometriosis. Fertil Steril. Jun 1998;69(6):1048-1055.

17. Redwine DB. Diaphragmatic endometriosis: diagnosis, surgical management, and long-term results of treatment. Fertil Steril. Feb 2002;77(2):288-296.

18. Slasky BS, Siewers RD, Lecky JW, Zajko A, Burkholder JA. Catamenial pneumothorax: the roles of diaphragmatic defects and endometriosis. AJR Am J Roentgenol. 1982;138(4):639-43.

19. Alifano M, Venissac N, Mouroux J: Recurrent pneu- mothorax

associated with thoracic endometriosis. Surg Endosc 2000; 14:680.

20. Alifano M, Roth T, Broet SC, Schussler O, Magdeleinat P, Regnard JF: Catamenial pneumothorax: A prospec- tive study. Chest 2003; 124:1004-1008.

21. Roth T, Alifano M, Schussler O, Magdaleinat P, RegnardJF: Catamenial pneumothorax: chest X-ray sign and thoracoscopic treatment. Ann Thorac Surg 2002; 74: 563-565.

22. Korom S, Canyurt H, Missbach A. Catamenial pneumothorax revisited: clinical approach and systematic review of the literature. J Thorac Cardiovasc Surg. 2004;128:502–8.

23. Alifano M. Catamenial pneumothorax. Curr Opin Pulm Med. 2010 Jul;16(4):381-6.

24. Mikroulis DA, Didilis VN, Konstantinou F, Vretzakis GH, Bougioukas GI. Catamenial pneumothorax. Thorac Cardiovasc Surg. 2008;56(6):374-5.

25. Korom S, Canyurt H, Missbach A, et al. Catamenial pneumothorax revisited: clinical approach and systematic review of the literature. J Thorac Cardiovasc Surg. Oct 2004;128(4):502-508.

26. Rossi NP, Goplerud CP. Recurrent catamenial pneumothorax. Arch Surg. Aug 1974;109(2):173-176.

27. Leong AC, Coonar AS, Lang-Lazdunski L, Catamenial pneumothorax: surgical repair of the diaphragm and hormone treatment. Ann R Coll Surg Engl. 2006;547-9.

28. Laws HL, Fox LS, Younger JB, Bilateral catamenial pneumothorax. Arch Surg. 1977;627-8.

29. Fonseca P., Catamenial pneumothorax: a multifactorial etiology. J Thorac Cardiovasc Surg. 1998;872-3.

30. Nezhat C, Nicoll L, Bhagan L, Huang J, Bosev D, Hajhosseini B, Beygui R. Endometriosis of the diaphragm: four cases treated with a combination of laparoscopy and thoracoscopy. J Minim Invasive Gynecol. 2009; 16(5)573-580-84..

31. Joseph J, Sahn SA, Thoracic endometriosis syndrome: new observations from an analysis of 110 cases. Am J Med. 1996;164-70.

32. Alifano M, Roth T, Broet SC, Schussler O, Magdeleinat P, Regnard JF. Catamenial pneumothorax: a prospective study. Chest. Sep 2003;124(3):1004-1008.

33. Joseph J, Sahn SA. Thoracic endometriosis syndrome: new observations from an analysis of 110 cases. Am J Med. Feb 1996;100(2):164-17012.

34. Jubanyik KJ, Comite F. Extrapelvic endometriosis. Obstet Gynecol

Clin North Am. Jun 1997;24(2):411-440.

35. Alifano M, Roth T, Broët SC, Catamenial pneumothorax: a prospective study. Chest. 2003;1004-8.

36. Alifano M, Jablonski C, Kadiri H, Catamenial and noncatamenial, endometriosis-related or nonendometriosis-related pneumothorax referred for surgery. Am J Respir Crit Care Med. 2007;1048-53.

37. Alifano M., Catamenial pneumothorax. Curr Opin Pulm Med. 2010;381-6.

38. Rousset-Jablonski C, Alifano M, Plu-Bureau G, Catamenial pneumothorax and endometriosis-related pneumothorax: clinical features and risk factors. Hum Reprod. 2011;2: 322-9.

39. Alifano M, Legras A, Rousset-Jablonski C, Pneumothorax recurrence after surgery in women: clinicopathologic characteristics and management. Ann Thorac Surg. 2011;322-6.

40. Van Schil PE, Vercauteren SR, Vermeire PA, Catamenial pneumothorax caused by thoracic endometriosis. Ann Thorac Surg. 1996;585-6.

41. Bagan P, Le Pimpec Barthes F, Assouad J, et al. Catamenial pneumothorax: retrospective study of surgical treatment. Ann Thorac

Surg 2003;75:378-81;

42. Morcos M, Alifano M, Gompel A, Life-threatening endometriosis-related hemopneumothorax. Ann Thorac Surg. 2006;726-9.

43. Alifano M, Trisolini R, Cancellieri A, Regnard JF. Thoracic endometriosis: current knowledge. Ann Thorac Surg. Feb 2006;81(2):761-769.

44. Nezhat CR BG, Nezhat F, Buttram VC Jr., Nezhat CH. Endometriosis: Advanced Management and Surgical Techniques. New York: Springer-Verlag.

45. Nezhat C, Seidman DS, Nezhat F. Laparoscopic surgical management of diaphragmatic endometriosis. Fertil Steril. Jun 1998;69(6):1048-1055.

46. Redwine DB. Diaphragmatic endometriosis: diagnosis, surgical management, and long-term results of treatment. Fertil Steril. Feb 2002;77(2):288-296.

47. Slasky BS, Siewers RD, Lecky JW, Zajko A, Burkholder JA. Catamenial pneumothorax: the roles of diaphragmatic defects and endometriosis. AJR Am J Roentgenol. 1982;138(4):639-43.

48. Marshall MB, Ahmed Z, Kucharczuk JC, Kaiser LR, Shrager JB. Catamenial pneumothorax: optimal hormonal and surgical management.

Eur J Cardiothorac Surg. Apr 2005;27(4):662-666.

49. Korom S, Canyurt H, Missbach A, et al. Catamenial pneumothorax revisited: clinical approach and systematic review of the literature. J Thorac Cardiovasc Surg. 2004;128(4):502-508.

50. Alifano M, Trisolini R, Cancellieri A, Regnard JF. Thoracic endometriosis: current knowledge. Ann Thorac Surg. Feb 2006;81(2):761-769.

51. Alifano M. Catamenial pneumothorax. Curr Opin Pulm Med. 2010 ; 16(4):381-6.

52. Hilaris GE, Payne CK, Osias J, Cannon W, Nezhat CR. Synchronous rectovaginal, urinary bladder, and pulmonary endometriosis. JSLS. Jan-Mar 2005;9(1):78-82.

53. Nezhat CR BG, Nezhat F, Buttram VC Jr., Nezhat CH. Endometriosis: Advanced Management and Surgical Techniques. New York: Springer-Verlag.

54. Camran Nezhat, Babak Hajhosseini, Elizabeth Buescher, Asrafjah Hussein, Georgios E. Hilaris, Michal Sellin Thoracic Endometriosis Syndrome.

55. Hilaris GE, Payne CK, Osias J, Cannon W, Nezhat CR. Synchronous rectovaginal, urinary bladder, and pulmonary endometriosis. JSLS. Jan-

Mar 2005;9(1):78-82.

56. Nezhat CR BG, Nezhat F, Buttram VC Jr., Nezhat CH. Endometriosis: Advanced Management and Surgical Techniques. New York: Springer-Verlag.

57. Kuo PH, Wang HC, Liaw YS, Kuo SH. Bronchoscopic and angiographic findings in tracheobronchial endometriosis. Thorax. Oct 1996;51(10):1060-1061.

58. Tabbara SO, Covell JL, Abbitt PL. Diagnosis of endometriosis by fine-needle aspiration cytology. Diagn Cytopathol. 1991;7(6):606-10.

59. Nezhat C, Nicoll L, Bhagan L, Huang J, Bosev D, Hajhosseini B, Beygui R. Endometriosis of the diaphragm: four cases treated with a combination of laparoscopy and thoracoscopy. J Minim Invasive Gynecol. Sept/Oct 2009; 16(5)573-580.

60. Nezhat C, Seidman DS, Nezhat F. Laparoscopic surgical management of diaphragmatic endometriosis. Fertil Steril. Jun 1998;69(6):1048-1055.

61. Augoulea A, Lambrinoudaki I, Christodoulakos G. Thoracic Endometriosis Syndrome. Respiration 2008; 75: 113-119.

62. Rafay M, El-Bawab H, Kurdli W, Al Kattan K. Diaphragmatic

fenestrations in catamenial pneumothorax: a management strategy. Asian Cardiovasc Thorac Ann 2009; 17: 70-72.

63. Alifano M, Trisolini R, Cancellieri A, Regnard JF. Thoracic endometriosis: current knowledge. Ann Thorac Surg 2006; 81: 761-769.

64. Flieder DB, Moran CA, Travis WD, Koss MN, Mark EJ. Pleuro-pulmonary endometriosis and pulmonary ectopic deciduosis: a clinicopathologic and immunohistochemical study of 10 cases with emphasis on diagnostic pitfalls. Hum Pathol 1998; 29: 1495-1503

65. Tabbara SO, Covell JL, Abbitt PL. Diagnosis of endometriosis by fine-needle aspiration cytology. Diagn Cytopathol. 1991;7(6):606-10.

66. Marshall M, Ahmed Z, Kucharczuk J. Catamenial pneumothorax: optimal hormonal and surgical management. Eur J Cardiothorac Surg. 2005;27:662–6.

7 ENDOMETRIOSIS AND MALIGNANCY

Endometriosis has mixed traits of benign disease and malignancy. The pathogenesis involves loss of control of cell proliferation and is associated with local and distant spread; however, endometriosis does not cause catabolic disturbance, metabolic consequences, or death [1-2]. Although endometriosis cannot be termed a premalignant condition, epidemiologic, histopathologic, and molecular data suggest that endometriosis does have malignant potential [1].

Epidemiology

There is suggestion regarding association between endometriosis and ovarian tumor. The suggestion is of a common mechanism based on similar disease responses, such as the protective effects of tubal ligation, hysterectomy, oral contraceptives, and pregnancy, increased risks with infertility, and early menarche, late menopause, and nulliparity for both ovarian cancer and endometriosis [1, 3]. The prevalence of ovarian cancer developing in women with endometriosis is higher than sporadic ovarian cancer in the general population [1].

Brinton et al., 1997 [4], reviewed 20,686 women hospitalized with endometriosis identified through the Swedish Inpatient Registry from 1969 to 1983 with a mean follow-up of 11.4 years. The cases of all incident cancers identifying 738 overall malignancies and 29 ovarian malignancies. Standardized incidence ratios (SIRs) with 95% confidence intervals (CIs) from this study showed an increased overall cancer risk of 1.2, 1.9 for ovarian cancer, 1.3 for breast cancer, and 1.8 for hematopoetic cancers [1,4].

Borgfeldt and Andolf 2004 [5], also identified a cohort of 28,163 endometriosis patients born before 1970 from the National Swedish Hospital Discharge Registry from 1969 to 1996 and matched each case with three controls. The cohort of endometriosis patients had an increased risk for ovarian cancer of 1.3 with a significantly lower mean age at diagnosis of 49 years versus 51.6 years in control population [1, 5].

Brinton et al.,2004 [6] did a retrospective cohort study conducted in the United States, analyzing the correlation of endometriosis causing primary infertility and ovarian cancer, resulting in an SIR of 4.19 and a risk ratio of 2.72 compared with patients with secondary infertility and no endometriosis [1, 6].

Another study from Japan [7] followed a cohort of 6,398 women with clinically documented endometriomas and evaluated the risk of ovarian cancer based on varying time periods from time of diagnosis of endometriosis [1, 7].

Few large retrospective series have evaluated the prevalence of ovarian malignancy among patients operated for endometriosis [8]. Mostoufizadeh and Scully reported eight cancers in 950 cases (0.8%) of ovarian endometriosis [8-9]. A similar prevalence (0.9%) has been documented by

Stern et al. in a series of 1000 patients with the disease [8, 13]. This latter prevalence raised to 3.8% if "arising in" was defined according to Sampson's criteria only, thus without the histological demonstration of a contiguity between the two entities [8, 11-12]

Whether or not endometriosis should be considered a preneoplastic disease represents a major and controversial issue [8]. Similarly to its eutopic uterine counterpart, studies on the epithelial lining of cystic ovarian endometriosis have documented the presence of metaplastic, hyperplastic, or atypical changes. The precise prevalence of these alterations in endometriosis and their significance in terms of risk to undergo malignant transformation are not defined [8, 13-15]. The data suggested that carcinoma may arise from endometriosis through a multi-step phenomenon where typical endometriosis may change into severe atypia with or without hyperplasia and then into carcinoma [8]. Studies prospectively evaluating the risk of cancer in patients with endometriotic atypia and/or complex hyperplasia are extremely scarce and inconclusive [8, 14,16-17].

Since endometriosis is associated with infertility, association between the disease and cancer should be interpreted with caution since an increased risk may be due to nulliparity rather than to endometriosis per se [8]. This bias may be particularly relevant for ovarian and breast cancer. Venn et al., 1999 [18], evaluated the incidence of gynecologic malignancies in a cohort of 29,700 infertile women using data from 10 Australian infertile clinics. The authors failed to observe an increased risk of breast cancer (SIR = 1.0; 95% CI, 0.7–1.5). The recruited sample size did not allow reliable analysis for uterine and ovarian cancers [8, 18].

Brunson et al., 1988 [19], described two cases of adenocarcinoma arising in extraovarian endometriosis 19 and 8 years following abdominal hysterectomy and bilateral salpingo-oophorectomy. Both patients presented with hydronephrosis. One had been on chronic estrogen therapy. The literature is reviewed in reference to frequency, tumor type, and sites of occurrence [19].

Reimnitz, et al, 1988 [20] presented two cases of malignancy arising from a dormant focus of endometriosis after total abdominal hysterectomy, bilateral salpingo-oophorectomy, and exogenous estrogen replacement therapy. These malignancies are often well differentiated and may behave similarly to estrogen-induced endometrial carcinomas. After removal of the ovaries of a premenopausal woman with endometriosis, the use of progestins in replacement therapy may reduce the risk of malignancy arising in endometriosis [20].

Zanetta, G. M., M. J. Webb, et al 2000 [21] studied the condition of hyperestrogenism (either endogenous or exogenous) which may cause hyperplasia or transformation into cancer. They studied retrospectively the patients who had tumors from endometriosis diagnosed from 1986 to 1997 Each patient was matched with two control patients (endometriosis without cancer) treated during the same study interval. Clinical and epidemiologic variables were compared to identify risk factors for the development of cancer. They found that hyperestrogenism, either endogenous or exogenous, is a significant risk factor for the development of cancer from endometriosis. The prevalences of endometriosis, obesity, and use of hormonal replacement therapy in women in developed countries are increasing, and this trend justifies the assumption that cancer developing in endometriosis might become more common in the future [21].

Epidemiological studies have shown that women with endometriosis have an increased risk of different types of malignancies, especially ovarian cancer and non-Hodgkin's lymphoma [22-24]. Nevertheless, other reports show also an association between endometriosis, dysplastic nevi, and melanoma, and breast cancer [22, 25-27].

Other less common sites include the rectovaginal septum, rectum, and sigmoid colon [28]. Endometrioid carcinoma is a common malignant tumour arising from endometriosis followed by clear cell carcinoma [28-30]

A case of Endometrial stromal sarcoma patient with extrauterine endometriosis has been reported [31]. A survey of 45 extragonadal malignancies associated with endometriosis in 1977 found that 16 (36%) were in the rectovaginal area, 5 (11%) in the colorectal area, 4 (9%) each in the bladder and vagina, 3 (7%) in the pelvic ligaments, and 2 (4%) each in the umbilicus, cervix, and fallopian tube [32]. A more recent survey of 27 malignancies associated with endometriosis found that 17 (62%) were in the ovary, 3 (11%) in the vagina, 2 (7%) each in the fallopian tube or mesosalpinx, pelvic sidewall, and colon, and 1 (4%) in the parametrium [28, 33].

Pathogenesis

Concerning ovarian cancer, several studies have indicated endometriosis as a risk factor and various histological and molecular genetic studies have indicated that endometriosis may transform into cancer [22, 34-38]. By microsatellite analysis, it has been recently demonstrated that loss of heterozygosity on p16(Ink4), GALT, and p53, as well as on APOA2, a region frequently lost in ovarian cancer, occurs in endometriosis, even in stage II of the disease. The occurrence of such genomic alterations may represent, therefore, important events in the development of endometriosis.

Moreover, the 9p21 locus where p16 is mapped, may contain a gene associated with the pathogenesis of the disease, and its loss may be a prognostic marker of the disease [22, 39].

Despite the histological and epidemiological evidence linking endometriosis and ovarian cancer, it is still not clear if endometriosis is a real precursor of ovarian cancer, or whether there is an indirect link involving common environmental, immunological, hormonal or genetic factors [40]. It has been clearly demonstrated that activation of a mutated K-ras gene is a fundamental step in the genesis and progression of ovarian cancer [41-42]. Moreover, it has been proposed that aberrant transcriptional regulation of the H-ras proto-oncogene is caused by p53 protein alterations: in fact, the human c-H-ras1 gene contains within the first intron a p53 element, which functions as a transcriptional enhancer [22, 43].

Dinulescu et al 2005 [44] have engineered a new transgenic mouse both as model of endometriosis and as a model of endometrioid ovarian carcinoma [38]. Briefly, by taking advantage of the Cre recombinase technology, Dinulescu et al 2005, [44] first generated mice with a mutationally activated K-ras gene: these mice developed spontaneously benign endometrioid lesions on the ovarian epithelium in all mice and peritoneal endometriosis in about half of the cases. In the second phase, these mice were engineered to lack the expression of Pten. This second mutation caused the insurgence of invasive endometrioid carcinomas of the ovary. This model represents the first mouse model of spontaneous human endometriosis and strongly suggests that the endometriotic lesions are initiated by endometrium refluxed through the fallopian tubes into the peritoneal cavity [22].

The association between endometriosis and epithelial ovarian carcinoma (EOC) has been supported by years of epidemiologic research [45]. The current knowledge of this association at the molecular level remains an area of great interest and worthy of future studies as the carcinogenic mechanisms and pathways remain poorly defined. Future studies will clarify the roles of oxidative stress, inflammation and estrogen in the development of endometriosis associated ovarian cancer (EAOC). At this point, we know that the micro-environment of endometriosis and EAOC share similar cytokines and mediators. Whether this similarity represents a link between endometriosis and EAOC or simply an employment of common signaling molecules to two separate lesions remains to be seen. Studies evaluating the possible intermediary lesion of EAOC (both contiguous and "atypical" endometriosis) appear promising in strengthening the link between endometriosis and ovarian carcinoma. These studies may also aid in identifying endometriotic lesions at greatest risk of malignant transformation. However, most of the specimens harboring these features are in formalin-fixed, paraffin-embedded (FFPE) form, which presents a challenge for successful molecular profiling and analysis. A greater understanding of the pathogenesis of EAOC would potentially allow for preventative strategies for those women with endometriosis at greatest risk of developing EAOC, as well as novel treatment approaches for women already diagnosed with EAOC [45].

The histopathological and epidemiological evidence demonstrating the strong association between endometriosis and ovarian cancer is given in the following subsections [46]. There are two hypotheses that could explain the link: (i) endometriotic implants may directly undergo malignant transformation, perhaps through an atypical endometriosis transition phase; and (ii) both endometriosis and cancer share common antecedent mechanisms and/or predisposing factors (e.g. genetic susceptibility, immune/ angiogenic dysregulation, environmental toxin exposure), with obvious divergence in molecular pathways downstream [46].

Morphometric analysis of cancer, used for assessing mitotic activity and grading, has been shown to correlate with clinical prognosis [47]. Although morphometric analysis of non-atypical endometriosis showed no difference between active (red) and inactive (black or white) lesions, it has yet to be studied in atypical endometriosis [48]. Nonetheless, mild cytological atypia in the glandular epithelium of endometriotic cysts has been associated with normal DNA diploid patterns, whereas severe atypia may be associated with aneuploidy [46, 49].

Pathological angiogenesis, immune cell suppression and immune cell activation co-exist in endometriosis and cancer processes [50]. Genetically transmitted or environmentally induced (e.g. exposure to dioxins) alterations in the angiogenic and/or immune response may predispose women to the ectopic implantation of endometrial cells, transported into the peritoneal cavity by retrograde menstruation, which thereby leads to endometriosis. Significantly, both cancer and endometriosis share some of the mediators implicated in this 'inflammatory angiogenesis' model. Furthermore, the genes of these mediators exhibit genetic polymorphisms that predispose either to endometriosis (e.g. intercellular adhesion molecule-1, IL-6 and IL-10 gene promoters) [51-52] or to cancer (e.g. IL-6, IL-8, tumour necrosis factor (TNF)-a, NFkB-1, and peroxisome proliferator-activated receptor-g genes) [46, 53].

Indeed there is extensive clinicopathological, molecular and genetic evidence supporting the hypothesis that endometriosis is a neoplastic process with a potential for malignant transformation [46]. Like sporadic cancer [54], endometriosis may be considered to arise by complex interactions between inherited germline polygenic low-penetrance alleles (polymorphisms) [55], somatically acquired genetic alterations, environmental factors [56]. Acceptance of this hypothesis permits the use of investigative strategies that have proved successful in defining the molecular processes that underlie cancer: genomic, transcriptomic and proteomic profiling [46]. Thus the analysis of genetic changes associated with normal endometrium, non-atypical, atypical and EAOC lesions could define the sequential changes involved in the initiation, proliferation and malignant transformation of endometriosis [46].

References

1. Farr Nezhat, M. Shoma Datta, Veneta Hanson, Tanja Pejovic, Ceana Nezhat, and Camran Nezhat. The relationship of endometriosis and ovarian malignancy: a review. Fertility and Sterility 2008; 90 (5): 1559-1570.

2. Thomas EJ, Campbell IG. Evidence that endometriosis behaves in a malignant manner. Gynecol Obstet Invest 2000;50(Suppl 1):2–10.

3. Van Gorp T, Amant F, Neven P. Vergote. Endometriosis and the development of malignant tumors of the pelvis. A review of literature. Best Pract Res Clin Obstet Gynaecol 2004;18:349–71.

4. Brinton LA, Gridley G, Persson I, Baron J, Bergqvist A. Cancer risk after a hospital discharge diagnosis of endometriosis. Am J Obstet Gynecol 1997;176:572–9.

5. Borgfeldt C, Andolf E. Cancer risk after hospital discharge diagnosis

of benign ovarian cysts and endometriosis. Acta Obstet Gynecol Scand 2004;83:395–400.

6. Brinton LA, Lamb EJ, Moghissi KS, Scoccia B, Althius MD, Mabie JE, Westhoff CL. Ovarian cancer risk associated with varying causes of infertility. Fertil Steril 2004;82:405–14.

7. Kobayashi H, Sumimoto K, Moniwa N, Imai M, Takakura K, Kuromaki T, et al. Risk of developing ovarian cancer among women with ovarian endometrioma: a cohort study in Shizuoka, Japan. Int J Gynecol Cancer 2007;17:37–43.

8. Edgardo Somigliana, Paola Vigano, Fabio Parazzini, Sandra Stoppelli, Erika Giambattista, Paolo Vercellini. Association between endometriosis and cancer: A comprehensive review and a critical analysis of clinical and epidemiological evidence. Gynecologic Oncology 2006; 101: 331 – 341.

9. Mostoufizadeh H, Scully RE. Malignant tumours arising in endometriosis. Clin Obstet Gynecol 1980; 23:951– 63.

10. Stern RC, Dash R, Bentley RC, Snyder MJ, Haney AF, Robboy SJ. Malignancy in endometriosis: frequency and comparison of ovarian and extraovarian types. Int J Gynecol Pathol 2001; 20:133– 9.

11. Sampson JA. Endometrial carcinoma of the ovary arising in endometrial tissue in that organ. Arch Surg 1925;10:1–72.

12. Scott RB. Malignant changes in endometriosis. Obstet Gynecol 1953;2:283– 9.

13. Fukunaga M, Nomura K, Ishikawa E, Ushigome S. Ovarian atypical endometriosis: its close association with malignant epithelial tumours. Histopathology 1997;30:249– 55.

14. Prefumo F, Todeschini F, Fulcheri E, Venturini PL. Epithelial abnormalities in cystic ovarian endometriosis. Gynecol Oncol 2002;84:280–4.

15. Czernobilsky B, Morris WJ, Seidman JD, Feeley KM, Wells M. A histologic study of ovarian endometriosis with emphasis on hyperplastic and atypical changes. Obstet Gynecol 1979;53:318– 23.

16. Seidman JD, Feeley KM, Wells M. Prognostic importance of hyperplasia and atypia in endometriosis. Int J Gynecol Pathol 1996;15:1– 9.

17. Fukunaga M, Ushigome S. Epithelial metaplastic changes in ovarian endometriosis. Mod Pathol 1998;11:784– 8.

18. Venn A, Watson L, Bruinsma F, Giles G, Healy D. Risk of cancer after use of fertility drugs with in-vitro-fertilization. The Lancet 1999;354:1586– 90.

19. Brunson, G. L., D. L. Barclay, et al. Malignant extraovarian

endometriosis: two case reports and review of the literature. Gynecol Oncol 1988; 30(1): 123 30.

20. Reimnitz, C., E. Brand, et al. Malignancy arising in endometriosis associated with unopposed estrogen replacement. Obstet Gynecol 1988; 71(3 Pt 2): 444-7.

21. Zanetta, G. M., M. J. Webb, et al. Hyperestrogenism: a relevant risk factor for the development of cancer from endometriosis. Gynecol Oncol 2000; 79(1): 18-22.

22. Alfonso Baldi, Mara Campioniand Pietro G. Signorile. Endometriosis: Pathogenesis, diagnosis, therapy and association with cancer (Review). Oncology Reports 2008; 19: 843-846.

23. Olson JE, Cerhan JR, Janney CA, Anderson KE, Vachon CM and Sellers TA: Postmenopasual cancer risk after self-reported endometriosis diagnosis in the Iowa women's health study. Cancer 2002; 94: 1612-1618.

24. Melin A, Sparen P and Bergqvist A: Endometriosis and the risk of cancer with special emphasis on ovarian cancer. Hum Reprod 2006; 21: 1237-1242.

25. Wyshak G, Frisch RE, Albright NL, Albright TE and Schiff I: Reproductive factors and melanoma of the skin among women. Int J Dermatol 1989; 28: 527-530.

26. Hornstein MD, Thomas PP, Sober AJ, Wyshak G, Albright NL and Frisch RE: Association between endometriosis, dysplastic nevi and history of melanoma in women of reproductive age. Hum Reprod 1997; 12: 143-145.

27. Bertelsen L, Mellemkjer L, Frederiksen K, Kyer SK, Brinton LA, Sakoda LC, van Valkengoed I and Olsen JH: Risk for breast cancer among women with endometriosis. Int J Cancer 2997; 120: 1372-1375.

28. Agarwal N, Subramanian A. Endometriosis - Morphology, clinical presentations and molecular pathology. J Lab Physician 2010; 2:1–9.

29. Scully RE, Young RH, Clement PB. Washington DC: Armed Forces Institute of Pathology; 1998. Endometrioid tumors In: Tumors of the ovary, maldeveloped gonads, fallopian tube, and broad ligament; pp. 107–40.

30. Scully RE, Young RH, Clement PB. Washington DC: Armed Forces Institute of Pathology; 1998. Clear cell tumors In: Tumors of the ovary, maldeveloped gonads, fallopian tube, and broad ligament; pp. 141–52.

31. Park Soo-Kyung, Sun-Joo Lee, Han Sung Kwon, In Sook Sohn, Ji Young Lee, Soo Nyung Kim, et al. Endometrial stromal sarcoma associated with extrauterine endometriosis: a case report and literature review. Kore J Gynecol Oncol. 2008;19:87–92.

32. Brooks JJ, Wheeler JE. Malignancy arising in extragonadal

endometriosis: a case report and summary of the world literature. Cancer. 1977;40:3065–73.

33. Leiserowitz GS, Gumbs JL, Oi R, Dalrymple JL, Smith LH, Ryu J, et al. Endometriosis-related malignancies. Int J Gynecol Cancer. 2003;13:466–71.

34. Melin A, Sparen P and Berqvist A: The risk of cancer and the role of parity among women with endometriosis. Hum Reprod 2997; 22: 3021-3026.

35. Ogawa S, Kaku T, Amada S, Kobayashi H, Hirakawa T, Arioshi K, Kamura T and Nakano H: Ovarian endometriosis associated with ovarian carcinoma: a clinicopathological and immunohistochemical study. Gynecol Oncol 2000; 77: 298-304.

36. Yoshikawa H, Jimbo H, Okada S, Matsumoto K, Onda T, Yasugi T and Taketani Y: Prevalence of endometriosis in ovarian cancer. Gynecol Obstet Invest 2000; 50: 11-17.

37. Varma R, Rollason T, Gupta JK and Maher ER: Endometriosis and the neoplastic process. Reproduction 2004; 127: 293-304.

38. Prowse AH, Manek S, Varma R, Liu J, Godwin AK, Maher ER, Tomlinson IPM and Kennedy SH: Molecular genetic evidence that endometriosis is a precursor of ovarian cancer. Int J Cancer 2006; 119: 556-562.

39. Goumenou AG, Arvanitis DA, Matalliotakis IM, Koumantakis EE and Spandidos DA: Microsatellite DNA assays reveal an allelic imbalance in p16(Ink4), GALT, p53, and APOA2 loci in patients with endometriosis. Fertil Steril 2001; 75: 160-165.

40. Ness RB, Grisso JA, Cottreau C, Klapper J, Vergona R, Wheeler JE, Morgan M and Schlesselman JJ: Factors related to inflammation of the ovarian epithelium and risk of ovarian cancer. Epidemiology 2000; 11: 111-117.

41. Mammas IN, Zafiropoulos A and Spandidos DA: Involvement of the ras genes in female genital tract cancer: Int J Oncol 2005; 26: 1241-1255.

42. Dokianakis DN, Varras MN, Papaefthimiou M, Apostolopoulou J, Simiakaki H, Diakomanolis E and Spandidos DA: Ras gene activation in malignant cells of human ovarian carcinoma peritoneal fluids. Clin Exp Metastasis 1999; 17: 293-297.

43. Zachos G and Spandidos DA: Transcriptional regulation of the c-H-ras1 gene by the P53 protein is implicated in the development of human endometrial and ovarian tumours. Oncogene 1998; 16: 3013-3017.

44. Dinulescu DM, Ince TA, Quade BJ, Shafer SA, Crowley D and Jacks T: Role of K-ras and Pten in the development of mouse models in endometriosis and endometrioid ovarian cancer. Nat Med 2005; 11: 63-

70.

45. Michael J. Worley Jr., William R. Welch, Ross S. Berkowitz and Shu-Wing Ng. Endometriosis-Associated Ovarian Cancer: A Review of Pathogenesis. Int. J. Mol. Sci. 2013; 14: 5367-5379.

46. Rajesh Varma, Terrance Rollason, Janesh K Gupta and Eamonn R Maher. Endometriosis and the neoplastic process. Reproduction 2004; 127: 293–304.

47. Kronqvist P, Kuopio T, Jalava P & Collan Y. Morphometrical malignancy grading is a valuable prognostic factor in invasive ductal breast cancer. British Journal of Cancer 2002; 87: 1275–1280.

48. Regidor PA, Wagner I, Ruwe M, Regidor M & Schindler AE. Morphometric analyses of endometriotic tissues to determine their grade of activity. Gynecological Endocrinology 2002; 16: 235–243.

49. Ballouk F, Ross JS & Wolf BC. Ovarian endometriotic cysts. An analysis of cytologic atypia and DNA ploidy patterns. American Journal of Clinical Pathology 1994; 102: 415–419.

50. Folkman J. Role of angiogenesis in tumor growth and metastasis. Seminars in Oncology 2002; 29 (Suppl 16):15–18.

51. Kitawaki J, Obayashi H, Ohta M, Kado N, Ishihara H, Koshiba H, Kusuki I, Tsukamoto K, Hasegawa G, Nakamura N, Yoshikawa T &

Honjo H. Genetic contribution of the interleukin-10 promoter polymorphism in endometriosis susceptibility. American Journal of Reproductive Immunology 2002; 47: 12–18.

52. Wieser F, Fabjani G, Tempfer C, Schneeberger C, Sator M, Huber J & Wenzl R. Analysis of an interleukin-6 gene promoter polymorphism in women with endometriosis by pyrosequencing. Journal of the Society for Gynecologic Investigation 2003; 10:32–36.

53. Landi S, Moreno V, Gioia-Patricola L, Guino E, Navarro M, de Oca J, Capella G & Canzian F. Association of common polymorphisms in inflammatory genes interleukin (IL)6, IL8, tumor necrosis factor alpha, NFKB1, and peroxisome proliferator-activated receptor gamma with colorectal cancer. Cancer Research 2003; 63: 3560–3566.

54. Balmain A, Gray J & Ponder B. The genetics and genomics of cancer. Nature Genetics 2003; 33 (Suppl): 238–244.

55. Zondervan KT, Cardon LR & Kennedy SH. The genetic basis of endometriosis. Current Opinion in Obstetrics and Gynecology 2001; 13: 309–314.

56. Birnbaum LS & Cummings AM. Dioxins and endometriosis: a plausible hypothesis. Environmental Health Perspectives 2002; 110: 15–21.

8 DIAGNOSIS OF ENDOMETRIOSIS

Introduction

Several studies have reported large diagnostic delays in endometriosis [1]. Recent studies report, specifically for Europe, an overall diagnostic delay of 10.4 years in Germany and Austria [2], 8 years in the UK and Spain [3-4], 6.7 years in Norway [3], 7–10 years in Italy and 4–5 years in Ireland and Belgium [4]. In these studies, several causes for this delay in diagnosis were suggested, including intermittent use of contraceptives causing hormonal suppression of symptoms, the use of non-discriminatory examinations, misdiagnosis, attitude towards menstruation and normalisation of pain by the women, their mothers, family doctors, gynecologists or other specialists [1-4].

Diagnostic strategy

There are no sufficiently sensitive and specific signs and symptoms or diagnostic tests for the clinical diagnosis of endometriosis, and no diagnostic strategy is supported by evidence of effectiveness [5]. The American College of Obstetricians and Gynecologists recommends a pretreatment diagnostic strategy to exclude other causes of pelvic pain such as chronic pelvic inflammatory disease, fibroid tumors, and ovarian cysts [6]. Nongynecologic causes of pain also should be excluded [5].

Pelvic and rectal examinations should be performed, although the yield of the physical examination is low. Findings of a retroverted uterus, decreased uterine mobility, cervical motion tenderness, and tender uterosacral nodularity are suggestive of endometriosis when present, but these findings often are absent. Laboratory tests and radiologic examinations usually are not warranted. Measurement of CA 125 levels may be useful for monitoring disease progress, and MRI has a high sensitivity in detecting endometrial cysts but poor diagnostic accuracy for endometriosis in general. Empiric diagnosis and treatment of endometriosis is reasonable, based on clinical suspicion and presentation. Patients with persistent symptoms after empiric treatment should be referred for laparoscopy, the preferred method for diagnosis of endometriosis [6].

Radiology:

Because symptoms of endometriosis are variable, patients may be referred for a diverse array of imaging studies, including excretory urography, barium studies, and computed tomography (CT) [7]. These techniques lack both sensitivity and specificity, and a variety of nonspecific radiologic findings may be seen [7].

a. Ultrasonography

Ultrasonography (US) is the most common imaging modality used to evaluate suspected endometriosis. However, it is applicable only to the evaluation of endometriotic cysts [7]. Both transvesicular and transvaginal US should be performed [7].

Endometriomas can have a variety of US appearances. The majority exhibit diffuse low-level internal echoes, with the "classic" endometrioma being described as a homogeneous, hypoechoic focal lesion within the ovary [7]. In one study of 40 endometrial cysts, 95% demonstrated this finding [8]. In rare cases, they may be anechoic, mimicking a functional ovarian cyst.

Endometriomas may be unilocular or multilocular. A multilocular-appearing endometrioma may actually consist of multiple separate cysts. Thin or thick septations may be present between these loculi. One study showed that in the absence of wall nodularity and in the presence of diffuse low-level echoes, a multiloculated mass was 64 times more likely to be an endometrioma [7-8].

The US appearance of the endometrial cyst wall can be variable but deserves special attention. Diffuse wall thickening, wall nodularity, and echogenic foci within the cyst wall have been observed [7-9].

Pelvic ultrasonography by the transvaginal route is reliable (NP2) and is most often sufficient to confirm or exclude the diagnosis of ovarian endometrioma (grade B). During transvaginal pelvic ultrasonography, care should be taken to explore the area located in front of the uterus and the retrocervical area [10].

In women with an adnexal mass with a suspicion of endometriosis, several studies were performed to evaluate the accuracy of TVS in ovarian endometriosis diagnosis [1]. In a systematic review, transvaginal and transabdominal ultrasound scanning (with or without Doppler) was evaluated as a diagnostic test for pelvic endometriosis. A total of 1257 adnexal masses were evaluated; histology was used in all but eight cases, where only cytology was performed. The prevalence of endometriosis was 13 to 38%. Diagnostic characteristics were: sensitivity 64 to 89%, specificity 89 to 100%, LR+ 7.6 to 29.8, and LR− 0.1 to 0.4 [1,11]. It has to be noted that women with ovarian endometriosis have more pelvic and intestinal areas invaded by endometriosis, compared to women without ovarian endometriosis [1,12]. Ovarian endometrioma are only rarely sole findings. This implies that if an ovarian endometrioma is diagnosed by TVS, attention should be given to the possible existence of deep infiltrating disease; this should be further investigated by performing thorough vaginal and rectovaginal examinations and, where indicated, by more extensive imaging techniques like MRI [1].

In cases where there is a strong suspicion of endometriosis, especially in deep infiltrating disease, studies have been performed to evaluate the accuracy of transvaginal sonography (TVS) to diagnose rectal endometriosis [1]. In a systematic review, the diagnostic value of TVS for non-invasive, pre-surgical detection of bowel endometriosis was evaluated in 1105 women. In all but 32 women, histological verification (the gold standard) was obtained where diagnosis was made by laparoscopic visualisation. In the studies evaluated, the prevalence (95% CI) of bowel endometriosis was 47% (36.7–57.3). In these studies, the following characteristics were found for TVS diagnosis of bowel endometriosis: sensitivity 91% (88.1–93.5); specificity 98% (96.7–99.0); LR+ 30.36 (15.457–59.626); LR– 0.09 (0.046–0.188); PPV 98% (96.7–99.6); NPV 95% (92.1–97.7) [1-2].

3D Sonography: The value of 3D sonography in detecting the presence of rectovaginal endometriosis was evaluated in a case series of 39 women with a clinical suspicion of rectovaginal endometriosis [1,13].

The prevalence of rectovaginal endometriosis was 50%, the investigators found: sensitivity (95% CI) 89.5% (73.3–94.5), specificity 94.7% (78,6–99,7), LR+ 17.2 (2.51–115) and LR– 0.11 (0.03–0.41) [1,13].

Perineal ultrasonography shows irregular hypoechoic mass in the perineal region with rounded or oval anechoic areas in it [14]. With some patients of Perineal endometriosis (PEM), the examination shows a heterogeneous mass containing cystic anechoic and hyperechoic areas. Perineal ultrasonography can help in the diagnosis of the lesion, but it fails in revealing the involvement of anal sphincter. Preoperative endoanal ultrasonography, on the contrary, is a reliable technique for visualizing perianal endometriosis and for diagnosing anal sphincter involvement. The ultrasonographic features of the lesion are similar to those mentioned above [14]. Its advantage over perineal ultrasonography is that it can reveal the involvement of anal sphincter clearly. Besides, endoanal ultrasonography can also help in the differential diagnosis of perianal lesions: ultrasonography of perianal abscess shows homogeneous hypoechoic lesions; ultrasonography of perianal fistula shows hypoechoic fistula passes through the longitudinal muscle tissues; ultrasonography of anal carcinoma and melanoma show solid lesions. As 16.7% of patients with PEM are concomitant with pelvic endometriosis, pelvic examination and pelvic ultrasonography should be taken to exclude pelvic endometriosis [14-17]

b. MR Imaging

Magnetic resonance (MR) imaging has proved to be a very useful and more specific imaging technique and is often used as a problem-solving tool [7]. MR imaging has been shown to have greater specificity for the diagnosis of endometriomas than other noninvasive imaging techniques [7, 18-21]. It affords a larger field of view than US, and the effect of adhesions on surrounding anatomic structures is better depicted [7].

Imaging planes can include all three standard projections (axial, sagittal, and coronal), with the sagittal plane being particularly useful for evaluating the cul-de-sac and rectum [7]. Endometriomas have a relatively homogeneous high signal intensity (similar to or greater than that of fat) on T1-weighted images.

Looking at both the multiplicity and signal intensity of lesions, Togashi et al [18], found that a "definitive" diagnosis of an endometrioma was made when a cyst was hyperintense on T1- weighted images and shading was observed on T2-weighted images. The diagnosis was also "definitive" when multiple hyperintense cysts were seen on T1-weighted images regardless of their signal intensity on T2-weighted images [7].

MR imaging yielded an overall sensitivity, specificity, and accuracy of 90%, 98%, and 96%, respectively. Because these cysts contain blood products of different ages and concentrations, cyst appearance can be variable. Those lesions that are not hyperintense on T1-weighted images can be difficult to distinguish from other adnexal masses [7, 18, 21].

Despite advances in technology, the diagnosis of small endometriotic implants remains elusive. Their signal intensity is quite variable. They may appear similar to normal endometrium (ie, low signal intensity on T1-weighted images and high signal intensity on T2-weighted images), be hypointense with all pulse sequences, or be hyperintense with all pulse sequences [7, 19, 21-22].

The value of magnetic resonance imaging (MRI) in detecting the presence of peritoneal endometriosis was evaluated by Stratton and co-workers [23] in a case series of 44 women with a clinical suspicion of endometriosis [1]. The prevalence of endometriosis was 86%, sensitivity was 69%, specificity was 75%, LR+ was 2.76, and LR− was 0.41. These LRs are too low to justify use of MRI to diagnose or exclude peritoneal disease. Overall, compared with biopsy results for each lesion, MRI had a diagnostic sensitivity of 38% and specificity of 74% [1, 23]. MRI is not useful to diagnose or exclude peritoneal endometriosis. Furthermore, the authors noted that MRI is not a cost-effective diagnostic tool [1, 23]

Imaging techniques such as computerized tomography (CT) scan, or MRI can identify cysts and help characterize the fluid within an ovarian cyst, although an endometriotic cyst and a normal corpus luteum cyst may have a similar appearance. These tests are useful when evaluating women experiencing infertility and/or chronic pelvic pain [24].

MRI provides the means of mapping the exact location of deep retroperitoneal lesions (NP2). It can thus be used as part of the preoperative workup, but systematic use is not recommended (consensus of professional opinion). It is useful where there is clinical suspicion of grade B. However, MRI is not generally recommended for the diagnosis of endometriomas [10].

Laparoscopy

Laparoscopy is the standard of reference in the diagnosis of endometriosis. Staging of the disease can also be done during laparoscopy [7]. Endometriotic implants, endometriomas, and adhesions are the typical findings. Implants may measure from a few millimeters to a few centimeters and may be superficial or deep [7]. Because endometriotic implants can vary in appearance, the accuracy of diagnosis depends on the ability of the surgeon to recognize the disease [7, 25]. A pattern of lesion maturity has been described, with subtle findings seen in young women and more characteristic features identified in the same women a decade later [7, 26].

Endometriotic cysts may be seen, most commonly involving the ovaries. Inflammatory response to active endometrial lesions can lead to fibrosis and adhesions. Severe adhesions may actually compartmentalize the pelvis and impede laparoscopic evaluation [7].

A systematic review on the accuracy of laparoscopy to diagnose endometriosis (with biopsy and histology as the gold standard) showed that only limited reports of good quality exist, when assessing the value of visual diagnosis of endometriosis at laparoscopy [1]. The accuracy of a diagnostic laparoscopy for endometriosis was evaluated in 433 patients. A negative diagnostic laparoscopy seems to be highly accurate for excluding endometriosis and is therefore of use to the clinician in aiding decision-making. However, a positive laparoscopy is less informative and of limited value when used in isolation (without histology); the positive likelihood ratio (LR+) (95% CI) is 4.30 (2.45–7.55), and the negative likelihood ratio (LR−) is 0.06 (0.01–0.47). With a prevalence of 20% the post-test probability is 51.8 (38.0–65.4) if the test is positive and 1.5 (0.2 10.5) if the test is negative [1,27]

Retroperitoneally and vaginally localized endometriosis can be easily missed, especially if the patient has not been thoroughly examined preoperatively, preferably during anesthesia [1].
Laparoscopy with or without histological verification is widely used to diagnose and rule out the presence of endometriosis. However, the literature on the diagnostic value of a laparoscopy is very limited [1, 27]

Endometriotic lesions identified visually at laparoscopy or laparotomy is the gold standard of diagnosis (grade A) [10]. Diagnostic laparoscopy for suspected endometriosis should be preceded by an appropriate workup. Endometriosis can give rise to many different types of lesions. Diagnostic laparoscopy may overlook certain endometriotic lesions, in particular deep retroperitoneal endometriotic lesions. The operation report must describe the size, macroscopic appearance, location and depth of infiltration for all the lesions, as well as the adhesions [10].

LABORATORY DIAGNOSIS

As endometriosis can be progressive in up to 50% of women [28-29], early noninvasive diagnosis has the potential to offer early treatment and prevent progression [28]. Transvaginal ultrasound (TVU) is an adequate diagnostic method to detect ovarian endometriotic cysts but does not rule out peritoneal endometriosis, endometriosis-associated adhesions [30-31], or some locations of deep infiltrating endometriosis (DIE) [32-34]. Furthermore, routine vaginal examination alone may be insufficient to detect endometriosis before laparoscopy [35-36]. A noninvasive test would be particularly welcome; recent evidence suggests that significant biologic differences exist between eutopic endometrium from women with and without endometriosis [37], so this may offer a basis for a semi-invasive diagnostic test based on the analysis of an endometrial biopsy sample [28].

Despite extensive research, no reliable blood tests currently exist for the diagnosis of endometriosis[28]. A biomarker is a measurable ''biologic marker'' that correlates with a specific outcome or state of the disease [38]. The biomarker hypothesis states that changes in levels of analytes, proteins, microRNA (miRNA), genes, or other markers could be a specific characteristic of the disease state [38]. Although CA-125, cytokines, and angiogenic and growth factors all show altered levels in the peripheral blood of women with endometriosis when compared with controls [39-40], thus far neither a single biomarker nor a panel of biomarkers has been validated for clinical use as a diagnostic test in women with endometriosis [40-41]. The development of a noninvasive diagnostic test—from initial biomarker discovery to a clinically approved biomarker assay—is a long, difficult, and uncertain process [28, 42].

A noninvasive test for endometriosis would be useful for women with pelvic pain and/or subfertility with normal ultrasound results. This would include nearly all cases of minimal-to-mild endometriosis, some cases of moderate to severe endometriosis without clearly visible ovarian endometrioma, and women with pelvic adhesions and/or other pelvic pathology, which might benefit from surgery to improve their pelvic pain and/or subfertility [28,36].

A noninvasive diagnostic test could be developed for serum, plasma, urine, or menstrual fluid that can be recovered from the posterior vaginal fornix or the cervix during speculum examination [28]. A semi-invasive test could be developed for peritoneal fluid obtained via transvaginal ultrasound–guided aspiration or for endometrium obtained via transcervical endometrial biopsy [28]. Whatever method is used, the most important goal of the test is that no women with endometriosis or other significant pelvic pathology are missed who might benefit from surgery [36]. To achieve this goal, a test with a high sensitivity is needed, which is the probability of a test of being positive when endometriosis is present. In addition, the test needs to have a high specificity, to ensure a high probability of the test being negative when endometriosis is absent [28]. Sensitivity and specificity are statistical measures of performance of a binary classification test, which could be a confounder in data analyses [28]. The predictive value of any diagnostic test is influenced by its sensitivity and specificity as well as the prevalence of the target disease in the population being evaluated. Thus, the predictive value of a diagnostic test includes information about both the test itself and the tested population to give a more useful clinical measure [28, 43-44]. A rule of thumb is that the sensitivity and specificity of a good test should add to at least 1.50, and those of a very good test should add to at least 1.80 [44-45]. At present, such a test does not exist [28, 30]. Although CA-125, cytokines, angiogenic and growth factors are differentially expressed in the peripheral blood of women with endometriosis when compared with controls [39-40, 46].

So far neither a single biomarker nor a panel of biomarkers has been validated as a non-invasive test for endometriosis [40], possibly because most studies included limited numbers of patients and limited assessment of different cycle phases and endometriosis stages [40]. Studies evaluating a panel of biomarkers [47] are also limited with respect to the number of biomarkers analysed, the statistics used (univariate statistical analysis) and the lack of validation in an independent test set of patients [46].

A biomarker that is easy to measure may possibly help clinicians to diagnose (or at least exclude) endometriosis; it might also help monitor the outcome of treatment. An effective marker or a panel of markers could help avoid needless diagnostic procedures and/or recognize treatment failure at an early stage. QUADAS (Quality Assessment of Diagnostic Accuracy Studies) criteria were applied to carry out a systematic review of the literature over the last 25 years with a view to evaluate seriously the clinical connotation of all proposed biomarkers for endometriosis in serum, plasma and urine. Of more than 100 putative biomarkers that satisfied the selection criteria they failed to identify a single biomarker or panel of biomarkers that have indisputably been shown to be clinically valuable peripheral biomarkers show promise as diagnostic aids, but further research is necessary before they can be recommended in routine clinical care. Panels of markers may permit increased sensitivity and specificity of any diagnostic test [48].

K.E. May et al 2011 [49], have reviewed the current accessible literature on endometrial differences in women with endometriosis, and evaluate their possible value as disease biomarkers. They used QUADAS (Quality Assessment of Diagnostic Accuracy Studies) criteria for a methodical review of published papers over the past 25 years and the search encompassed all studies assessing differences between eutopic endometrium of women with and without endometriosis. The review identified 182 relevant articles evaluating more that 200 potential biomarkers, including hormones and their receptors ($n = 29$), cytokines ($n = 25$), factors identified using proteomics ($n = 8$) and histological analysis ($n = 10$) of endometrial tissue. Sensitivity and specificity were reported or could be calculated for only 32 articles, and ranged from 0 to 100%., six of the nine topmost quality studies identified biomarkers related to nerve fibre growth or cell cycle control. The review recognized several reports of endometrial differences which have the promise of biomarkers of endometriosis, larger studies in well-defined populations are undoubtedly warranted to verify their exact value.

A study was conducted to compare the density of multiple-sensory small-diameter nerve fibres in endometrium from women with endometriosis and those without endometriosis. The study enrolled 40 women with confirmed minimal–mild endometriosis and 20 women without endometriosis. Immunohistochemistry was performed to localize neural markers for sensory C, Aδ, adrenergic and cholinergic nerve fibres in the functional layer of the secretory phase endometrium. Sections were immunostained with anti-human protein gene product 9.5

(PGP9.5), anti-neurofilament protein, anti-substance P (SP), anti-vasoactive intestinal peptide (VIP), anti-neuropeptide Y and anti-calcitonine gene-related polypeptide. The density of small nerve fibres was ~14 times higher in endometrium from patients with minimal–mild endometriosis (1.96 ± 2.73) in comparison with normal women Immunohistochemistry was performed to localize neural markers for sensory C, Aδ, adrenergic and cholinergic nerve fibres in the functional layer of the secretory phase endometrium. Sections were immunostained with anti-human protein gene product 9.5 (PGP9.5), anti-neurofilament protein, anti-substance P (SP), anti-vasoactive intestinal peptide (VIP), anti-neuropeptide Y and anti-calcitonine gene-related polypeptide. The density of small nerve fibres was ~14 times higher in endometrium from patients with minimal–mild endometriosis when compared with normal women The combined analysis of neural markers PGP9.5, VIP and SP could forecast the presence of minimal–mild endometriosis with 95% sensitivity, 100% specificity and 97.5% accuracy. , Prospective studies are recommended to confirm their findings [50].

Paucity of a non-invasive diagnostic test accounts for protracted delay between the start of symptoms and diagnosis of endometriosis. A control study was conducted to assess the individual performance of a panel of six selected plasma biomarkers in the diagnosis of endometriosis .The study enrolled 294 infertile women, comprising 93 normal women and 201 women with endometriosis. It showed increased plasma levels of IL-6, IL-8 and CA-125 in all women with endometriosis and in those with minimal–mild endometriosis, relative to controls. In women with moderate–severe endometriosis, plasma levels of IL-6, IL-8 and CA-125, and hsCRP, were considerably elevated as compared to controls. Advanced statistical analysis of the panel of six selected plasma biomarkers on samples obtained during the secretory phase or during menstruation helps in the diagnosis of all stages with high sensitivity and clinically acceptable specificity [47].

a. Known Biomarkers

1. **Interleukin-6 (IL-6)** is a T cell-derived cytokine that is secreted by macrophages, lymphocytes, fibroblasts, and endothelial cells. It has B cell stimulatory activity and enhances the differentiation of T lymphocytes [51-52]. IL-6 secretion is increased by peritoneal macrophages in endometriosis patients and by stromal cells of eutopic and ectopic endometrium, with the ectopic stromal cells producing the highest levels [51, 53]. IL-6 normally inhibits the growth of endometrial cells; however, this growth-inhibitory effect is lost in endometriotic tissues [51, 54]. It has been found that serum IL-6 to provide the best discrimination between subjects with endometriosis and healthy controls [51].

2. **Monocyte chemotactic protein-1 (MCP-1)** is produced by T cells, monocytes, and endometrial cells, and it plays an important role in the recruitment of monoytes and macrophages to the peritoneal cavity in subjects with endometriosis [51-52]. MCP-1 is elevated in the peritoneal fluid of subjects with endometriosis, as compared with controls [51, 55-56]. Moreover, there is higher expression of MCP-1 in the eutopic and ectopic endometrium of subjects with endometriosis, where it is upregulated by the synergistic action of estradiol and IL-1b [51, 57]. It has been found that significantly elevated serum levels of MCP-1 in subjects with endometriosis compared with controls [51].

3. **Interferon-gamma INF-δ** regulates MCP-1 secretion by peripheral blood mononuclear cells [51, 58] and by endometriotic cells [51, 59]. In addition, INF-δ upregulates the expression of intracellular adhesion molecule-1 [51].

- Studies have examined serum cytokines as diagnostic markers for endometriosis; however, the results were conflicting. Bedaiwy et al 2002 [60]. found that serum IL-6 provides a sensitivity of 90% and a specificity of 67% for the diagnosis of endometriosis at a cutoff value of 2 pg/ml [51, 60]. Somigliana et al 2004 [61]. found no statistically significant difference in serum IL-6 concentration between subjects with endometriosis and controls; consequently, they could not recommend measuring IL-6 in the serum as a predictor of endometriosis [51, 61].

4. **T-plastin**, a cytoplasmic protein regulating actin assembly and cellular motility, is up-regulated in the secretory phase endometrium from women with minimal to mild endometriosis [62].

5. **Annexin V**, a calcium phospholipid-binding protein belonging to the annexin family, is up-regulated in secretory phase endometrium from women with minimal to mild endometriosis [62]. The role of annexin V in the pathogenesis of endometriosis is unclear, but, in cancer studies, annexin V is expressed exclusively in the periphery of invasively growing tumor areas, suggesting that it may play a role in proliferation and/or cell mobility and may have metastatic potential [63]. It has been hypothesized that annexin V plays a role in the early invasion of endometrial cells into the mesothelium after initial attachment to the peritoneal wall [62].

Panel of potential endometrial biomarkers including T-plastin and annexin V with a sensitivity of 100% and specificity of 100% for the diagnosis of minimal to mild endometriosis [62].

6. **Cancer antigen 125 (CA-125),** is widely used peripheral biomarker of endometriosis [28, 64], is produced by endometrial and mesothelial cells and gains entry into the circulation via the endothelial lining of capillaries in response to inflammation [65] However, CA-125 levels in peripheral blood lack diagnostic power as a single biomarker of

endometriosis due to low sensitivity [28, 65].

7. **Glycodelin**, is an endometrium-derived protein with known angiogenic, immunosuppressive, and contraceptive effects, could contribute to the development of endometriosis and endometriosis-related infertility [28, 66]. Increased plasma glycodelin levels have been observed in patients with endometriosis [28, 67-68].

8. **Vascular endothelial growth factor (VEGF)** is one of the main stimuli for angiogenesis and increased vessel permeability, contributes to the development of endometriotic lesions [28, 69-70]. However, there is no consensus regarding the value of VEGF as biomarker of endometriosis [28].

9. **Soluble intercellular adhesion molecule-1 (sICAM-1)** one of the major adhesion molecules that inhibits natural killer cell–mediated cytotoxicity [28, 71], resulting in defective immune surveillance, is involved in the implantation and development of endometriotic lesions [28, 72].

10. **Serum antiendometrial antibodies** [73]: Antiendometrial antibodies have been postulated to be a probable cause of infertility in endometriosis patients as shown by some investigators [74-75] but not by others [73, 76].

The sensitivity and the specificity of serum anti-endometrial antibodies screening were reported by some investigators to be 0.84 and 1.00, respectively [77]. On comparing infertile women with endometriosis with unexplained infertility, Wild and Shiver found a sensitivity of 0.71 and a specificity of 1.00 [73]. Similarly, Meek et al.[78] found a sensitivity of 0.75 and a specificity of 0.90 while in another study the values were 0.85 and 0.67, respectively [79]. Although serum antiendometrial antibodies matches CA 125 regarding both sensitivity and specificity, it does not satisfy the criteria of an ideal screening test. Despite this limitation, anti-endometrial antibody was proposed not only as a screening marker but as a follow-up marker of treatment results and recurrence as well [73, 80].

HISTOLOGY

Most patients with endometriosis have multiple sites of involvement. When histological diagnostic criteria are used, the ovaries are the most common site (36%) the fallopian tubes, uterus and cul-de-sac account for 6-14% of biopsies, and the uterosacral ligaments account only for 2% of specimens examined. On a clinical basis, 5-12% of women present extrapelvic endometriosis and in descending order in the sigmoid, the appendix, and omentum, on operative scars and in inguinal region. Rarely endometriosis is observed in distant sites such as lungs, brain, bones and skin [81-82].

Gross features of endometriosis

The location and the age of the endometriotic lesion and the patients' age affect the morphological appearance of endometriosis and may lead to diagnostic difficulties. Gross appearance of endometriotic lesions is affected by their age and this is reflected by the various colors they present. Red color characterizes early lesions and yellow-red color reflects the breakdown of blood products. These lesions eventually progress into old or advanced lesions presenting black color. Hemosiderin is indicated by a yellowish color and occasionally white lesions may be observed indicating the presence of fibrosis. It is possible that the same patient presents endometriotic foci in various stages of development. The size of the lesions varies as well. In early stages blister-like blebs are observed measuring 0.2-0.3 cms in diameter, corresponding to the early red lesion observed mainly in adolescents. As the lesions age, they may enlarge up to 1 cms in diameter and are pigmented, bluish-red, black and eventually white and puckered because of fibrosis. Endometriotic foci are frequently associated with adhesions. The older the patient the more fibrotic the endometriotic lesion is and eventually it atrophies with obliteration of its components. Endometriotic lesions become grossly cystic only in the ovaries reaching a diameter up to 15 cms. Ovarian endometriotic cysts present a fibrous wall of various thickness and are filled by chocolate-like contend. The interior surface may be smooth or shaggy. Rarely, endometriosis obtains the form of polypoid masses projecting from serosal surfaces and is referred as polypoid endometriosis [81].

Microscopic features of endometriosis

Endometriosis in women of reproductive age characteristically displays islands of one or more endometrioid glands with stromal cells around them; these resemble the endometrial stromal cells of the proliferative phase. The one layer thick glandular epithelium consists of cuboidal or columnar cells with eosinophilic cytoplasm and ovoid perpendicularly oriented nuclei; hardly any mitoses is present. The endometrial lining cells may have cilia and the stroma may show hyperemic vasculature. There may be decidual change in the stroma associated with the exogenous administration of progestins, or pregnancy. The stroma may display diffuse histiocytic infiltrate; presence of pseudoxanthoma cells originating from transformed histiocytes that have changed erythrocytes into glucolipid and brown pigment composed of lipofuscin and and some hemosiderin The density of pigment laden cells increase with the advancing age of the lesions. Inflammatory cells may be seen and some smooth muscle cells particularly in lining of the wall of endometrioid cysts. It is important to note that not all these may easily be noted.

Ovarian endometrioid cysts in particular appear to have stroma, with fibrosis, lined by hemosiderin-laden macrophages. In fact several histological sections may have to examine to identify the glandular component of endometriosis. It is important to bear in mind that macrophages may be related to hemorrhagic follicles or corpora lutea and diagnosis of endometriosis is based on the presence of glandular epithelium. The degree of cyclic changes of the glandular component depend on the amount of fibrous tissue, the amount of stroma round the glands, the degree of vascularity and the steroid receptor content. Endometriosis in places with native smooth muscle component may induce marked hypertrophy identical to that observed in cases of adenomyosis that leads to creation of adenomyomata or adenomyomatous nodules [81, 83].

It is important to record the possible changes one can come across while examining the histological profile of endometriosis. The glandual component of endometriosis may show metaplasia and hyperplastic changes. There may be metaplastic alterations include presence of ciliated, eosinophilic, clear cell, transitional cells and occasionally mucinous metaplasia usually of endocervical type. Hyperplasis of glandular epithelium may occur consequent to endogenous or exogenous hormonal action. These changes may mimic various grades of endometrial hyperplasia. In ovarian endometrioid adenocarcinoma one can detect remnants of endometriosis with hyperplastic changes. Likewise stromal metaplasia occur in the endometriotic stroma as well, of smooth muscle type. Simultaneous hyperplastic changes may result in endomyometriotic nodules or uterus–like masses, in the ovary, broad ligament, the bowel and lymph nodes

The glandular cells of endometriosis may present metaplastic changes such as ciliated, eosinophilic, clear cell and rarely squamous, transitional and rarely mucinous metaplasia usually of endocervical type. It is reported that in cases with extensive metaplastic changes in endometriosis an association with an ovarian epithelial tumor is observed. Glandular epithelium may present hyperplastic changes due to endogenous or exogenous hormonal action resembling hyperplastic endometrial changes from simple cystic to complex atypical hyperplasia. In cases of ovarian endometrioid adenocarcinoma remnants of endometriosis with hyperplastic changes are observed. Metaplastic changes are observed in the endometriotic stroma as well, of smooth muscle type. Concomitant hyperplastic changes may create endomyometriotic nodules or uterus–like masses, in the ovary, broad ligament, the bowel and lymph nodes [81].

The presence of stromal elements in the absence of glandular epithelium in foci of endometriosis constitutes the stromal endometriosis. This is encountered in the ovary, in the cervix and the peritoneum and usually is associated with a focus of typical endometriosis [81].

There are lesions known as necrotic pseudoxanthomatous nodules occur in postmenopausal women and are multiple nodules usually attached to peritoneum or floating free in the peritoneal cavity. They consist of a central fibrotic or hyalinized core with central necrosis surrounded by lipid laden histiocytes. Occasionally multiple sections will reveal remnants of endometriotic foci, and typical ovarian endometriosis co-exists [81].

Superficial cervical endometriosis is observed in the lamina propria of ectocervix as a solitary or multiple hemorrhagic nodules (endovervix is rarely involved by endometriosis) [81].

Neoplastic transformation of both the glandular and the stroma component of endometriosis may occur. There are benign and malignant lesions that may develop in endometriotic foci. Tumor-like benign lesions in the form of nodules or even larger, uterus-like masses are reported. Histological examination showed hyperplastic chances of the glandular component of endometriosis and extensive leiomyomatous metaplasia of the stromal component. These lesions may be described as endometrioid adenomas or endometrioid cystadenomas. Malignant transformation of the glandular component presents the pathological features of an endometrioid adenocarcinoma. In 75% of cases the malignant transformation of the glandular component arises in the ovaries [81]

Having outlined the histological profile of endometriosis it is essential to discuss briefly the problems in the diagnosis of endometriosis. The frequent problems in the differential diagnosis of endometriosis. In the majority of cases the microscopic features are typical and a diagnosis of endometriosis is easy. Nevertheless there may be problems because of metaplastic changes in the glands or when there is scarcity or absence of glands, as in stromal endometriosis [84]. Secondary changes of fibrosis with haemosiderin or lipofuscin deposition with effacement of glands or stroma may also occur, with consequent diagnostic difficulties [85]. Stromal decidual change occur in pregnancy or with progestagen therapy [3]. Stromal myxoid change in endometriosis has been infrequently reported [86-89] and many histopathologists may be unacquainted with this phenomenon, which is not described in standard pathology texts [90].

Other common problems in the differential diagnosis of endometriosis are briefly touched upon. Endometriotic cyst of the ovary may be confused with hemorrhagic follicle cysts or cystic corpora lutea.,however, the presence of granular layer cells or luteinized cells in the latter will resolve the diagnostic dilemma.The diagnosis of serosal inclusion cysts is determined by the lining of serous cells without any stromal component and related alterations. Rete ovarii with typical branching architecture and lacks stromal cells and haemorrhage can be diagnosed with ease. Mesonephric and paramesonephric remnants have a lining of low cuboidal epithelium enveloped by smooth muscle.Dermoid cysts which may have a lining composed of macrophages and granulation tissue can be diagnosed by the presence of squamous cells and hair fragments..

It is noteworthy that in cases that are laparoscopically diagnostic of endometriosis but the typical picture of endometriosis cannot be recognized and only stromal cells and other changes such as hemorrhage and macrophages are seen. In these cases the most appropriate diagnosis is that the lesion is "compatible with endometriosis" [81].

References

1. Management of women with endometriosis. Guideline of the European Society of Human Reproduction and Embryology. ESHRE Endometriosis Guideline Development Group September 2013.

2. Hudelist G, Fritzer N, Thomas A, Niehues C, Oppelt P, Haas D, Tammaa A and Salzer H. Diagnostic delay for endometriosis in Austria and Germany: causes and possible consequences. *Hum Reprod* 2012; **27**:3412–3416.

3. Ballard K, Lowton K and Wright J. What's the delay? A qualitative study of women's experiences of reaching a diagnosis of endometriosis. *Fertil Steril* 2006; 86:1296–1301.

4. Nnoaham KE, Hummelshoj L, Webster P, d'Hooghe T, de Cicco Nardone F, de Cicco Nardone C, Jenkinson C, Kennedy SH, Zondervan KT and World Endometriosis Research Foundation Global Study of Women's Health consortium. Impact of endometriosis on quality of life and work productivity: a multicenter study across ten countries. *Fertil Steril* 2011; 96:366–373.

5. Anne L. Mounsey, Alex Wilgus, David C. Slawson. Diagnosis and Management of Endometriosis. American Family Physician, 2006; 74

(4). Available at www.aafp.org/afp. Downloaded 20th March 2014.

6. ACOG Committee on Practice Bulletins—Gynecology. ACOG practice bulletin. Medical management of endometriosis. Number 11, December 1999 (replaces Technical Bulletin Number 184, September 1993). Clinical management guidelines for obstetrician-gynecologists. Int J Gynaecol Obstet 2000; 71:183-96.

7. Paula J. Woodward, Roya Sohaey, Thomas P. Mezzetti, Jr. From the Archives of the AFIP; Endometriosis: Radiologic-Pathologic Correlation. RadioGraphics 2001; 21:193–216.

8. Patel MD, Feldstein VA, Chen DC, Lipson SD, Filly RA. Endometriomas: diagnostic performance of US. Radiology 1999; 210:739–745.

9. Jain KA. Prospective evaluation of adnexal masses with endovaginal gray-scale and duplex and color Doppler US: correlation with pathologic findings. Radiology 1994; 191:63–67.

10. CNGOF Guidelines for the Management of Endometriosis Issued 29 nov, 2006- English translation M. Canis (2007)– Availble at www.cngof.asso.fr/D_TELE/RPC_endometriose_en_BM / Downloaded 25th March 2014.

11. Moore J, Copley S, Morris J, Lindsell D, Golding S and Kennedy S. A systematic review of the accuracy of ultrasound in the diagnosis of endometriosis. Ultrasound Obstet Gynecol 2002; 20:630–634.

12. Redwine DB. Ovarian endometriosis: a marker for more extensive pelvic and intestinal disease. Fertil Steril 1999; 72:310–315.

13. Pascual MA, Guerriero S, Hereter L, Barri-Soldevila P, Ajossa S, Graupera B and Rodriguez I. Diagnosis of endometriosis of the rectovaginal septum using introital three-dimensional ultrasonography. Fertil Steril 2010; 94:2761–2765.

14. Lan Zhu, Na Chen and Jinghe Lang (2012). Diagnosis and Treatment of Perineal Endometriosis, Endometriosis - Basic Concepts and Current Research Trends, Prof. Koel Chaudhury (Ed.), ISBN: 978-953- 51-0524-4, InTech, Available from: http://www.intechopen.com/books/endometriosis basic-concepts-andcurrent- research-trends/diagnosis-and-treatment-of-perineal-endometriosis. Downloaded 25th March 2014.

15. Bacher H, Schweiger W, Cerwenka H & Mischinger HJ. Use of anal endosonography in diagnosis of endometriosis of the external anal sphincter: report of a case. Dis Colon Rectum 1999; 42(5): 680-682.

16. T. Toyonaga, M. Matsushima & Y.Tanaka, et al. Endoanal ultrasonography in the diagnosis and operative management of perianal

endometriosis: report of two cases. Tech Coloproctol 2006; 10: 357-360.

17. Watanabe M, Kamiyama G & Yamazaki K, et al. (2003). Anal endosonography in the diagnosis and management of perianal endometriosis: report of a case. Surg Today 2003; 33: 630-632.

18. Togashi K, Nishimura K, Kimura I, et al. Endometrial cysts: diagnosis with MR imaging. Radiology 1991; 180:73–78.

19. Arrive L, Hricak H, Martin MC. Pelvic endometriosis: MR imaging. Radiology 1989; 171:687–692.

20. Dooms GC, Hricak H, Tscholakoff D. Adnexal structures: MR imaging. Radiology 1986; 158: 639–646.

21. Togashi K. Endometriosis. In: MRI of the female pelvis. Tokyo, Japan: Igaku-Shoin, 1993; 203–226.

22. Zawin M, McCarthy S, Scoutt LM, Comite F. Endometriosis: appearance and detection at MR imaging. Radiology 1989; 171:693–696.

23. Stratton P, Winkel C, Premkumar A, Chow C, Wilson J, Hearns-Stokes R, Heo S, Merino M and Nieman LK. Diagnostic accuracy of laparoscopy, magnetic resonance imaging, and histopathologic examination for the detection of endometriosis. Fertil Steril 2003; 79:1078–1085.

24. American Society for Reproductive Medicine. Endometriosis. A

Guide for Patients Revised 2012. Available at https://www.asrm.org/Endometriosis_booklet/ Accessed 25th March 2014.

25. Lu PY, Ory SJ. Endometriosis: current management. Mayo Clin Proc 1995; 70:453–463.

26. Redwine DB. Age related evolution in color appearance of endometriosis. Fertil Steril 1987; 48: 1062–1063.

27. Wykes CB, Clark TJ and Khan KS. Accuracy of laparoscopy in the diagnosis of endometriosis: a systematic quantitative review. BJOG 2004; 111:1204–1212.

28. Amelie Fassbender, Alexandra Vodolazkaia, Philippa Saunders, Dan Lebovic, Etienne Waelkens, Bart De Moor, and Thomas D'Hooghe. Biomarkers of endometriosis. Fertility and Sterility 2013; 99 (4): 1135-1145.

29. D'Hooghe TM, Debrock S. Endometriosis, retrograde menstruation and peritoneal inflammation in women and in baboons. Hum Reprod Update 2002;8:84–8.

30. Kennedy S, Bergqvist A, Chapron C, D'Hooghe T, Dunselman G, Greb R, et al. ESHRE guideline for the diagnosis and treatment of endometriosis. Hum Reprod 2005;20:2698–704.

31. Moore J, Copley S, Morris J, Lindsell D, Golding S, Kennedy S. A systematic review of the accuracy of ultrasound in the diagnosis of endometriosis. Ultrasound Obstet Gynecol 2002;20:630–4.

32. Dessole S, Farina M, Rubattu G, Cosmi E, Ambrosini G, Nardelli GB. Sonovaginography is a new technique for assessing rectovaginal endometriosis. Fertil Steril 2003;79:1023–7.

33. Bazot M, Thomassin I, Hourani R, Cortez A, Darai E. Diagnostic accuracy of transvaginal sonography for deep pelvic endometriosis. Ultrasound Obstet Gynecol 2004;24:180–5.

34. Bazot M, Lafont C, Rouzier R, Roseau G, Thomassin-Naggara I, Darai E. Diagnostic accuracy of physical examination, transvaginal sonography, rectal endoscopic sonography, and magnetic resonance imaging to diagnose deep infiltrating endometriosis. Fertil Steril 2009;92:1825–33.

35. Hudelist G, Ballard K, English J, Wright J, Banerjee S, Mastoroudes H, et al. Transvaginal sonography vs. clinical examination in the preoperative diagnosis of deep infiltrating endometriosis. Ultrasound Obstet Gynecol 2011; 37:480–7.

36. D'Hooghe TM, Mihalyi AM, Simsa P, Kyama CK, Peeraer K, De Loecker P, et al. Why we need a noninvasive diagnostic test for minimal to mild endometriosis with a high sensitivity. Gynecol Obstet Invest

2006;62:136–8.

37. Giudice LC, Kao LC. Endometriosis. Lancet 2004;364:1789–99.

38. Kingsmore SF. Multiplexed protein measurement: technologies and applications of protein and antibody arrays. Nat Rev Drug Discov 2006;5: 310–20.

39. Othman Eel D, Hornung D, Al-Hendy A. Biomarkers of endometriosis. Expert Opin Med Diagn 2008;2:741–52.

40. May KE, Conduit-Hulbert SA, Villar J, Kirtley S, Kennedy SH, Becker CM. Peripheral biomarkers of endometriosis: a systematic review. Hum Reprod Update 2010;00:1–24.

41. Vodolazkaia A, El-Aalamat Y, Popovic D, Mihalyi A, Bossuyt X, Kyama CM, et al. Evaluation of a panel of 28 biomarkers for the non-invasive diagnosis of endometriosis. Hum Reprod 2012;27:2698–711.

42. Surinova S, Schiess R, Huttenhain R, Cerciello F, Wollscheid B, Aebersold R. On the development of plasma protein biomarkers. J Proteome Res 2011; 10:5–16.

43. Friedland D. Evidence based medicine: a framework for clinical practice. New York: McGraw-Hill; 1998.

44. Sims JM. Clinical notes on uterine surgery. London: Robert Hardwicke; 1886.

45. Griffith CS, Grimes DA. The validity of the postcoital test. Am J Obstet Gynecol 1990;162:615–20.

46. A. Vodolazkaia, Y. El-Aalamat, D. Popovic, A. Mihalyi, X. Bossuyt, C.M. Kyama, A. Fassbender, et al. Evaluation of a panel of 28 biomarkers for the non-invasive diagnosis of endometriosis. Human Reproduction 2012; 0 (0): 1–14.

47. Mihalyi A, Gevaert O, Kyama CM, Simsa P, Pochet N, De Smet F, De Moor B, Meuleman C, Billen J, Blanckaert N et al. Non-invasive diagnosis of endometriosis based on a combined analysis of six plasma biomarkers. Hum Reprod 2010;25:654–664.

48. K.E. May, S.A. Conduit-Hulbert, J. Villar,S. Kirtley, S.H. Kennedy and C.M. Becker. Peripheral biomarkers of endometriosis: a systematic review Hum. Reprod 2010; 16 (6): 651-674.

49. K.E. May, J. Villar, S. Kirtley, S.H. Kennedy andC.M. Becker. Endometrial alterations in endometriosis: a systematic review of putative biomarkers Hum. Reprod. 2011; 17 (5): 637-653.

50. A. Bokor, C.M. Kyama, L. Vercruysse, A. Fassbender, O. Gevaert, A. Vodolazkaia, B. De Moor, V. Fülöp and T. D'Hooghe. Density of small diameter sensory nerve fibres in endometrium: a semi-invasive diagnostic test for minimal to mild endometriosis Hum. Reprod. 2009; 24 (12): 3025-3032.

51. Essam El-Din R. Othman, Daniela Hornung, Hosam T. Salem, Essam A. Khalifa, Tarek H. El-Metwally, Ayman Al-Hendy. Serum cytokines as biomarkers for nonsurgical prediction of endometriosis. European Journal of Obstetrics & Gynecology and Reproductive Biology 2008; 137:240–246

52. Ulukus M, Arici A. Immunology of endometriosis. Minerva Ginecol 2005; 57:237–48.

53. Berkkanoglu M, Arici A. Immunology and endometriosis. Am J Reprod Immunol 2003;50:48–59.

54. Dmowski WP, Braun DP. Immunology of endometriosis. Best Pract Res Clin Obstet Gynaecol 2004;18:245–63.

55. Akoum A, Lemay A, McColl S, Turcot-Lemay L, Maheux R. Elevated concentration and biologic activity of monocyte chemotactic protein-1 in the peritoneal fluid of patients with endometriosis. Fertil Steril 1996; 66(1):17–23.

56. Arici A, Oral E, Attar E, Tazuke SI, Olive DL. Monocyte chemotactic protein-1 concentration in peritoneal fluid of women with endometriosis and its modulation of expression in mesothelial cells. Fertil Steril 1997;67:1065–72.

57. Akoum A, Jolicoeur C, Boucher A. Estradiol amplifies interleukin-1-induced monocyte chemotactic protein-1 expression by ectopic

endometrial cells of women with endometriosis. J Clin Endocrinol Metab 2000;85:896–904.

58. Yoshimura T, Robinson EA, Tanaka S, Appella E, Leonard EJ. Purification and amino acid analysis of two human monocyte chemoattractants produced by phytohemagglutinin-stimulated human blood mononuclear leukocytes. J Immunol 1989;142:1956–62.

59. Akoum A, Lemay A, Brunet C, Hebert J. Cytokine-induced secretion of monocyte chemotactic protein-1 by human endometriotic cells in culture. The Groupe d'Investigation en Gynecologie. Am J Obstet Gynecol 1995;172(2 (Pt. 1)):594–600.

60. Bedaiwy MA, Falcone T, Sharma RK, et al. Prediction of endometriosis with serum and peritoneal fluid markers: a prospective controlled trial. Hum Reprod 2002;17:426–31.

61. Somigliana E, Vigano P, Tirelli AS, et al. Use of the concomitant serum dosage of CA 125, CA 19-9 and interleukin-6 to detect the presence of endometriosis. Results from a series of reproductive age women undergoing laparoscopic surgery for benign gynaecological conditions. Hum Reprod 2004;19:1871–6.

62. Cleophas M. Kyama, Attila Mihalyi, Olivier Gevaert, Etienne Waelkens, Peter Simsa, Raf Van de Plas, Christel Meuleman, Bart De Moor, and Thomas M. D'Hooghe. Evaluation of endometrial biomarkers

for semi-invasive diagnosis of endometriosis. Fertility and Sterility 2011; 95(4): 1338-1343

63. Melle C, Ernst G, Schimmel B, Bleul A, Koscielny S, Wiesner A, et al. Biomarker discovery and identification in laser microdissected head and neck squamous cell carcinoma with ProteinChip technology, two-dimensional gel electrophoresis, tandem mass spectrometry, and immunohistochemistry. Mol Cell Proteomics 2003;2:443–52.

64. Gupta S, Agarwal A, Sekhon L, Krajcir N, Cocuzza M, Falcone T. Serum and peritoneal abnormalities in endometriosis: potential use as diagnostic markers. Minerva Ginecol 2006; 58:527–51.

65. Mol BW, Bayram N, Lijmer JG, Wiegerinck MA, Bongers MY, van der Veen F, et al. The performance of CA-125 measurement in the detection of endometriosis: a meta-analysis. Fertil Steril 1998;70:1101–8.

66. Seppala MKH, Koistinen R, Hautala L, Chiu PC, Yeung WS. Glycodelin in reproductive endocrinology and hormone-related cancer. Eur J Endocrinol 2009;160:121–33.

67. Telimaa SKA, R€onnberg L, Suikkari AM, Sepp€al€a M. Elevated serum levels of endometrial secretory protein PP14 in patients with advanced endometriosis: suppression by treatment with danazol and high-dose medroxyprogesterone acetate. Am J Obstet Gyneacol

1989;161:866–71.

68. Koninckx PR, Riittinen L, Seppala M, Cornillie FJ. CA-125 and placental protein 14 concentrations in plasma and peritoneal fluid of women with deeply infiltrating pelvic endometriosis. Fertil Steril 1992;57:523–30.

69. Taylor RN, Lebovic DI, Mueller MD. Angiogenic factors in endometriosis. Ann NY Acad Sci 2002;955:89–100; discussion 118, 396–406.

70. Becker CM, D'Amato RJ. Angiogenesis and antiangiogenic therapy in endometriosis. Microvasc Res 2007;74:121–30.

71. Becker JCDR, Hartmann AA, Burg G, Schmidt RE. Schedding of ICAM-1 from human melanoma cell lines induced by INF-g and tumor necrosis factor alpha: functional consequence of cell-mediated cytotoxicity. J Immunol 1991;11:3788–93.

72. Wu MY, Ho HN. The role of cytokines in endometriosis. Am J Reprod Immunol 2003;49:285–96.

73. M. A. Bedaiwy, T. Falcone. Peritoneal fluid environment in endometriosis; Clinicopathological implications. Minerva Ginecologica 2003;55: 1-13.

74. Weed JC, Arquembourg PC. Endometriosis: can it produce an

autoimmune response resulting in infertility? Clin Obstet Gynecol 1980;23:885-93.

75. Badawy SZ, Cuenca V, Stitzel A, Jacobs RD, Tomar RH. Autoimmune phenomena in infertile patients with endometriosis. Obstet Gynecol 1984;63:271-5.

76. Dunselman GA, Bouckaert PX, Evers JL. The acutephase response in endometriosis of women. J Reprod Fertil 1988;83:803-8.

77. Mathur S, Peress MR, Williamson HO, Youmans CD, Maney SA, Garvin AJ *et al*. Autoimmunity to endometrium and ovary in endometriosis. Clin Exp Immunol 1982;50:259-66.

78. Meek SC, Hodge DD, Musich JR. Autoimmunity in infertile patients with endometriosis. Am J Obstet Gynecol 1988;158:1365-73.

79. Wild RA, Hirisave V, Podczaski ES, Coulam C, Shivers CA, Satyaswaroop PG. Autoantibodies associated with endometriosis: can their detection predict presence of the disease? Obstet Gynecol 1991;77:927-31.

80. Kennedy SH, Starkey PM, Sargent IL, Hicks BR, Barlow DH. Antiendometrial antibodies in endometriosis measured by an enzyme-linked immunosorbent assay before and after treatment with danazol and nafarelin. Obstet Gynecol 1990;75:914-8.

81. Agatha Kondi-Pafitis (2012). Pathological Aspects of Endometriosis, Endometriosis - Basic Concepts and Current Research Trends, Prof. Koel Chaudhury (Ed.), ISBN: 978-953-51-0524-4, InTech, Available from: http://www.intechopen.com/books/endometriosis-basic-concepts-and-current-research-trends/pathologicalaspects- of-endometriosis/ Downloaded 28th March 2014.

82. Jenkins S, Olive DL, Haney AF. Endometriosis: pathogenetic implications of the anatomic distribution. Obstet Gynecol 1986; 67:335-8.

83. Anaf V, Simon P, Fayt I, Noel J. Smooth muscles are frequent components of endometriotic lesions. Hum Reprod 2000; 15:767-71.

84. Clement PB, Young RH, Scully RE. Stromal endometriosis of the uterine cervix: a variant of endometriosis that may simulate a sarcoma. Am J Surg Pathol 1990; 14:449–55.

85. Clement PB, Young RH, Scully RE. Necrotic pseudoxan- thomatous nodules of ovary and peritoneum in endome- triosis. Am J Surg Pathol 1988; 12:390–7.

86. Clement PB, Granai CO, Young RH, et al. Endometriosis with myxoid change. A case simulating pseudomyxoma peritonei. Am J Surg Pathol 1994;18:849–53.

87. Nogales FF, Martin F, Linares J, et al. Myxoid change in

decidualised scar endometriosis mimicking malignancy.J Cutan Pathol 1993;20:87–91.

88. Hameed A, Jafri N, Copeland LJ, et al. Endometriosis with myxoid change simulating mucinous adenocarcinoma and pseudomyxoma peritonei. Gynecol Oncol 1996;62:317–19.

89. Ying AJ, Copeland LJ, Hameed A. Myxoid change in non-decidualised endometriosis resembling malignancy. Gyne- col Oncol 1998;68:301–3.

90. W G McCluggage, S J Kirk Pregnancy associated endometriosis with pronounced stromal myxoid change J Clin Pathol 2000;53:241–242 241

9 PHARMACOTHERAPY OF ENDOMETRIOSIS

RENU AGARWAL; PhD and NAFEEZA MOHD ISMAIL; PhD,

Faculty of Medicine, Universiti Teknologi MARA, 47000 Sungai Buloh, Selangor, Malaysia.

Treatment of endometriosis is challenging and involves surgical as well as medical therapies. Both the medical and surgical options have shown equal efficacy except for the treatment of infertility, which requires surgical options (Van Gorp et al. 2004). Pharmacological treatments act primarily by suppressing the ovulation and, therefore, fail to restore or maintain fertility (ACOG 1999; Hughes et al. 2007). Endometriosis causes appearance of symptoms 37% of the time in patients with mild disease and 74% of the time in those with severe disease (Winkel 2003). Although, the goal should be to eliminate the endometriotic lesions, more important is to treat the symptoms and prevent recurrences. Pharmacotherapy in endometriosis, therefore, primarily aims to provide symptomatic relief but has not been shown to be effective in preventing recurrence once the treatment is stopped.

The pharmacological treatment of endometriosis consists of non-steroidal anti-inflammatory drugs (NSAIDs), progestagens, combined oral contraceptive pills (COCPs), gonadotropin-releasing hormone (GnRH) analogues, antiprogestins, danazole, aromatase inhibitors, Selective Estrogen Receptor Modulators (SERMs) and Selective Progesterone Receptor Modulators (SPRMs).

NON-STEROIDAL ANTI-INFLAMMATORY DRUGS

Non-steroidal anti-inflammatory drugs (NSAIDs) are the first-line treatment for endometriosis related pain and remain the only medical option available for women attempting to conceive. They act as anti-inflammatory, antipyretic and analgesics by inhibiting the enzyme cyclooxygenase and, thereby inhibit the synthesis of pro-inflammatory mediators. The evidence to show that they are highly effective in relieving endometriosis related pain, however, remains inconclusive (Allen et al. 2009). The animal studies have indicated that NSAIDs like indomethacin and rofecoxib may also suppress the growth of endometrial implants. However, these findings have not been confirmed in human studies.

PROGESTAGENS

Progestagens are considered first line of treatment as their efficacy in relieving pain is comparable to danazole or GnRH analogues. They act by exerting a negative feedback on hypothalamus, hence causing a hypo-gonadotropic hypo-oestrogenic state and anovulation. Suppression of ovulation is the most important mechanism of pain relief by progestagens (Bulun 2009). Additionally, they cause decidualisation of the endometrium followed by its atrophy, hence exerting an anti-proliferative effect. However, the efficacy of progestagens in causing endometrial atrophy is less than that of danazole (Fedele et al. 1995). Progestagens also cause suppression of matrix metalloproteinases, which are involved in the implantation of the eutopic endometrium (Ferrero et al. 2010). Several progestagens are in use, however, there is no evidence that a particular progestagen at a particular dose is more effective than others. Commonly used progestagens and their ovulation inhibitory doses are listed in table 1.

Synthetic progestagens are rapidly absorbed after oral administration and reach the maximum serum concentration in 2-5 hours. In serum, they bind with sex hormone binding globulin (SHBG), cortisol binding globulin (CBG) or albumin. Many of them undergo metabolism in liver and are excreted in urine. Some of them are prodrugs and are metabolized in liver to active compounds; for example desogestrel to 3-keto-desogestrel and norgestimate to norgestrel.

Table 1: Commonly used progestagens and their ovulation inhibitory dose (Schindler et al. 2003)

Class	Progestagen	Ovulation inhibitory dose (mg/day; orally)
17α-Hydroxyprogesterone derivatives (pregnanes)	Medroxyprogesterone acetate	10
	Chlormadinone acetate	1.5-2
	Cyproterone acetate	1
19 nortestosterone derivatives	Norethindrone acetate	0.5
	Dienogest	1
Spirolactone derivative	Drospirenone	2
Retroprogesterone	Dydrogesterone	>30

The action of progestagens is mediated through intracellular steroid receptors known as progesterone receptors (PR), which are of two subtypes; PR-A and PR-B. Different progestagens vary in their affinity to PR as well as other steroid receptors and hence vary in their biological activity. Relative affinity of selected progestagens for PR and other steroid receptors is listed in table 2 and their biological activity is summarized in table 3. Medroxyprogesterone acetate, norethindrone acetate, cyproterone acetate and dienogest have been studied more widely and are discussed here.

Table 2: Relative affinity of various progestagens for steroid receptors and binding proteins (Schindler et al. 2003)

	PR	AR	ER	GR	MR	SHBG	CBG
MPA	115	5	0	29	160	0	0
Chlormadinone acetate	67	5	0	8	0	0	0
Cyproterone acetate	90	6	0	6	8	0	0
Norethindrone acetate	75	15	0	0	0	16	0
Dienogest	5	10	0	1	0	0	0
Drospirenone	35	65	0	6	230	0	0
Dydrogesterone	75	0	-	-	-	-	-

PR: progesterone receptor; AR: androgen receptor; ER: estrogen receptor; GR: glucocorticoid receptor; MR: mineralocorticoid receptor; SHGB: sex hormone-binding globulin; CBG: corticosteroid-binding globulin. The relative affinity is with reference to the following considered to have 100% affinity:

PR- Promegestone; AR- Metribolone; ER- estradiol-17β; GR-Dexamethasone;

MR- Aldosterone; SHBG- Dihydrotestosterone; CBG- Cortisol

Table 3: Biological activity of selected progestagens (Schindler et al. 2003)

	Progest agenic	Ant-GnRH	Anti-estro-geni c	Estro-genic	Andro-genic	Anti-andro-genic	Gluco-cortico id	Anti-miner corticoid
PA	+	+	+	-	±	-	+	-
hlormadino e acetate	+	+	+	-	-	+	+	-
yproterone etate	+	+	+	-	-	++	+	-
orethindron acetate	+	+	+	+	+	-	-	-
ienogest	+	+	±	±	-	+	-	-

spirenone	+	+	+	-	-	+	-	+
rogestero	+	-	+	-	-	±	-	±

(+) effective; (±) weakly effective; (−) not effective.

Medroxyprogesterone acetate (MPA) administered orally at a dose of 30-50 mg/day has been used to relieve endometriosis-associated pain since 1970s (Moghissi and Boyce 1976; Roland et al. 1976). Pain relief after treatment with a 50 mg/day dose of MPA for a short duration of 3 months is not more than that with placebo (Harrison and Barry-Kinsella 2000). However, when administered at a dose of 100 mg/day for 6 months, MPA is as effective as danazole in relieving pain after diagnostic laproscopy as well as after surgical excision (Telimaa et al. 1987a and 1987b). Administration of MPA for 6 months is also effective in relieving anxiety and depression. Improvement in the quality of life is comparable to GnRH analogues (Bergqvist and Theorell 2001).

Intramuscularly administered depot MPA (50 mg every 3 months) has also been used for pain relief and its efficacy after 1 year of treatment was found to be comparable to COCPs administered in combination with danazole (50 mg/day for 21 days in a 28 day menstrual cycle) (Vercellini et al. 1996). A subcutaneous formulation of depot MPA, 104 mg/0.65 ml (DMPA-SC 104), has also been found to be as effective as GnRH analogues in relieving pain (Crosignani et al. 2006a).

Orally administered MPA has 100% bioavailability as it does not undergo 1st pass metabolism and it does not bind with SHBG or CBG. Up to 88% of MPA in serum is bound to albumin.

Norethindrone acetate administered at a dose of 5-20 mg/day has been shown to be effective in relieving endometriosis-associated pain. At a low dose of 2.5 mg/day, it was shown to relive the pain in patients with rectovaginal endometriosis as effectively as estrogen-progesterone combination along with cyproterone acetate (Vercellini et al. 2005; Ferrero et al. 2009). Addition of norethindrone acetate (2.5 mg/day for 6 months) to on-going treatment with letrozole, an aromatase inhibitor, more effectively relieves pain compared to addition of triptorelin, a GnRH analog, (11.25 mg every 3 months, intramuscular) (Ferrero et al. 2009). Long-term use of norethindrone acetate for the treatment of recurrent endometrioma has also been shown to be effective in relieving pain and causing regression of cysts (Muneyyirci-Delale et al. 2012).

Norethindrone acetate is a unique progestin as it has both estrogenic and androgenic properties. To alleviate the hypoestrogenic symptoms associated with GnRH analogues, it can be used as an add-back regimen without estrogen supplementation because of its estrogenic properties. Additionally, it exerts beneficial effects on bone mineral density and vasomotor symptoms in women treated with GnRH analogues. However, it may lower high-density lipoprotein due to androgenic activity (Chwalisz et al. 2012). Bioavailability of orally administered norethindrone acetate is about 64%. In serum 36% is bound to SHBG and 61% to albumin.

Cyproterone acetate, a 17a-hydroxyprogesterone derivative, has been used as monotherapy in the treatment of endometriosis. It has antiandrogenic and antigonadotropic properties. After 6 months of treatment at a dose of 12.5 mg/day orally, cyproterone acetate has been shown to relieve endometriosis-associated pain as effectively as COCPs (Vercellini et al. 2002).

Orally administered cyproterone acetate is 100% bioavailable as it does not undergo 1st pass metabolism and is not bound to either SHBG or CBG, however, up to 93% is bound to serum albumin. It undergoes metabolism by hydroxylation and deacetylation. The metabolites have an antiandrogenic efficacy equivalent to that of cyproterone acetate, however the progestagenic activity is poor. It accumulates in fatty tissue and, therefore, administration of high daily doses causes depot effect due to accumulation.

Dienogest is an oral progestagen and is approved as monotherapy for endometriosis in Japan, Australia, Europe and Singapore. Dienogest at a dose of 2 and 4 mg/day has been shown to effectively relieve the endometriosis-associated pain. Both the doses have shown comparable efficacy and the adverse effects at these doses are generally tolerable (Köhler et al. 2010; Momoeda and Taketani 2007). When compared to placebo, dienogest 2 mg was shown to provide significantly greater pain relief (Strowitzki et al. 2010a). Randomized controlled trials have shown that dienogest 2 mg/day given for 16-24 weeks provides the pain relief, which is comparable to that produced by a GnRH analogue. However, the irregular bleeding is more frequent in dienogest group while the hot flushes are more frequent in GnRH group (Cosson et al. 2002; Harada et al. 2009; Strowitzki et al. 2010b). The efficacy, safety, and tolerability profile of dinogest has been shown to be favourable even when administered over an extended period of 65 weeks (Momoeda et al. 2009; Petraglia et al. 2012).

Orally administered dienogest is rapidly absorbed with a bioavailability of 90%. It does not bind with SHBG or CBG but 90% is bound to serum albumin and remaining exists as the free circulating form.

COMBINED ORAL CONTRACEPTIVE PILLS (COCPs)

COCPs have long been used in the empirical treatment of dysmenorrhea. They cause decidualisation of endometrial tissue and hence a state of "pseudopregnancy" and amenorrhea. This is followed by endometrial atrophy over several months. COCPs can be used continuously or cyclically. Besides oral, other dosage forms such as transdermal patches and vaginal rings are also available. The components of some of the commonly used COCPs are listed in table 4.

Table 4: The components of some of the commonly used COCPs (Halis et al. 2010)

Second generation	Third generation
Levonorgestrel 100 μg + Ethinyl estradiol 20 μg	Dienogest 2 mg + Ethinyl estradiol 30 μg EE
Levonorgestrel 150 μg + Ethinyl estradiol 30 μg EE	Norgestimate 250 μg + Ethinyl estradiol 35 μg EE
Levonorgestrel 250 μg + Ethinyl estradiol 30 μg	Gestodene 0.750 μg + Ethinyl estradiol 30 μg
Norethisterone 0.5 mg + Ethinyl estradiol 20 μg	Desogestrel 150 μg + Ethinyl estradiol 20 μg
Norethisterone acetate 0.5 mg + Ethinyl estradiol 30 μg	Desogestrel 150 μg + Ethinyl estradiol 30 μg

Norethisterone acetate 1.5 mg + Ethinyl estradiol 30 µg	Chlormadinone acetate 2 mg + Ethinyl estradiol 30 µg

The effectiveness of cyclical administration of low-dose monophasic COCPs (ethinylestradiol plus norethisterone) in relieving dysmenorrhea associated with endometriosis has been demonstrated in a placebo-controlled randomized double blind trial (Harada et al. 2008). The efficacy of these COCPs in cyclic regimen is comparable to GnRH analogues in relieving endometriosis-associated pain (Vercellini et al. 1993). Use of COCPs in cyclic regimen is also beneficial for prophylaxis against development or recurrence of endometriosis.

Administration of COCPs in continuous regimen may be more effective in patients presenting mainly with dysmenorrhea and in those undergone surgical excision (Seracchioli et al. 2009). Oral contraceptives taken continuously or in long cycles may be beneficial particularly for menstrual symptoms and the recurrence of symptoms (Hee et al. 2013). One of the randomized controlled trials has shown that daily administration of COCPs containing ethinyl estradiol 0.03 mg and gestodene 0.075 mg for 24 weeks provides significant pain relief in patients undergone conservative surgery. This efficacy of COCPs was comparable to intramuscular depot MPA (150 mg) every 12 weeks for 24 weeks (Cheewadhanaraks et al. 2012).

The adverse effects of COCPs are dose-dependent. Common adverse effects include nausea, edema, headache, bleeding, acne and hirsutism. The serious adverse effects of low dose COCPs are minimal in women without risk factors. Accordingly, in non-smokers without hypertension or diabetes, there is no significant increase in the risk of myocardial infarction or stroke. The risk of thrombosis increases with increasing dose particularly in women with predisposing risk factors such as smoking. In long-term users (>5 years) with persistent human papilloma virus infection, the risk of cervical carcinoma increases. High doses can also impair insulin sensitivity.

GONADOTROPIN-RELEASING HORMONE ANALOGUES

GnRH analogues play a leading role in the pharmacotherapy of endometriosis. They are modified forms of the native GnRH but have a longer half-life. They bind with the GnRH receptors in pituitary and cause initial stimulation and increased secretion of gonadotropins. This initial phase of stimulation lasts for 5-10 days and may temporarily exacerbate the symptoms. Continued administration, however, causes gonadotropin downregulation and suppression of ovarian steroid production. GnRH analogues therefore, rapidly induce a reversible hypo-oestrogenic state progressing to endometrial atrophy and amenorrhea similar to that of menopause and hence provide rapid relief from endometriosis-associated pain. They also relieve the symptoms of bladder and colorectal endometriosis. GnRH analogues are not effective in improving the endometriosis-associated infertility. However, their administration for 3-6 months before assisted reproductive technologies increase the odds of clinical pregnancy by at least four-fold (Sallam et al. 2006).

The GnRH analogues that are currently in use include leuprolide, nafarelin, histrelin, buserelin, goserelin and triptorelin. Numerous randomized controlled trials shown that the efficacy of GnRII analogues and their efficacy in relieving endometriosis-related pain is comparable to danazole, COCPs gestrinone, MPA and levonorgestrel intrauterine device (Fraser et al. 1991; Cirkel et al. 1995; Child et al. 2001; Bergqvist et al. 2001; Petta et al. 2005). No significant difference has been observed in the pain relieving efficacy of different GnRH analogues. Administration of GnRH analogues for 6 months to one year after operative laparoscopy has been shown to effectively relieve pain and prevent recurrence (Hornstein et al. 1997; Ferrero et al. 2007). However, postoperative GnRh therapy for shorter duration of 3 months is not as effective in relieving pain and preventing recurrence (Loverro et al. 2008).

GnRH analogues are inactive orally. They are administered as nasal spray, intramuscularly or subcutaneously. The injectable form is available as a short-acting preparation for daily use and a depot form to be used every 1-3 months. Commonly used GnRH analogues are listed in table 5.

Since GnRH analogues cause ovarian suppression, their use is associated with several hypo-estrogenic adverse effects. Short-term adverse effects include hot flushes, vaginal dryness, loss of libido, depression, joint pain, fatigue and emotional instability. Long-term use is associated with substantial loss of bone mineral density (BMD) after 12 months of continuous therapy, hence limiting the duration of therapy to 6 months.

In order to reduce the adverse effects and prolong the duration of treatment, "add-back" regimens in the form of small doses of steroid hormones are added if administration of GnRH analogues is required for more than 6 months. The add-back regimens generally consist of a progestagen, a combination of progesterone and oestrogen or progesterone combined with bisphosphonate. Commonly used regimens are listed in table 5. The amount of progesterone/oestrogen used as add-back therapy is sufficient to prevent the adverse effects due to hypo-estrogenic state but is lower than that required to produce stimulatory effect on endometriotic lesions (Barbieri 1998). Randomized controlled trials have demonstrated that add-back therapy does not reduce the efficacy of GnRH analogues but the short and long-term hypoestrogenic adverse effects are prevented (Franke et al. 2000). However, the high cost of GnRH analogues with add back therapy compared to progestagens and COCPs poses considerable limitation.

Table 5: GnRH analogues and add-back regimen (Crosignani et al. 2006b)

GnRH ANALOGUES		COMPONENTS OF ADD-BACK REGIMEN	
Drugs	Dose and administration	Regimen	Drugs (Duration of treatment)
Leuprolide	1 mg/day daily subcutaneous injection	Progesterone only	MPA (6 months)
			Norethindrone acetate (12 months)
Leuprolide depot	3.75 mg monthly intramuscular injection; 11.75 mg 3 monthly intramuscular injection		Norethindrone (12 months)
			Tibolone (6 months)

Triptorelin	3 mg monthly intramuscular injection	Progestin + bisphosphonate	Norethindrone + sodium etidronate (48 weeks)
Triptorelin depot	11.25 mg 3 monthly intramuscular injection	Progestin + estrogen	MPA + Conjugated equine estrogen (6 months)
Goserelin	3.6 mg subcutaneous implant monthly		MPA + 17β- estradiol (6 months)
			Norethindrone + 17β- estradiol (6 months)
Buserelin	300–400 μg intranasal thrice daily		Norethindrone acetate + Conjugated equine estrogen (12 months)
Nafarelin	200–400 μg intranasal twice daily		

GESTRINONE

Gestrinone is an antiprogestational 19-norsteroid derivative with antigonadotropic properties. It blocks the luteinizing hormone (LH) surge and limits the gonadotropin release. When administered orally at a dose of 2.5-10 mg daily or weekly for 6 months, its pain relieving efficacy is comparable to GnRH analogues (Gestrinone Italian Study Group 1996).

The uses of other progestagens such as lynestrenol, megestrol acetate, dydrogesterone, desogestrel have also been described. Use of an intrauterine device releasing levonorgestrel has been evaluated in women undergone operative laproscopy. The device was found to significantly reduce the medium-term risk of recurrence of moderate or severe dysmenorrhea (Vercellini et al. 2003). In a systematic review involving 3 randomized controlled trials, it was observed that the implant causes significantly greater reduction in the recurrence of painful periods compared to expectant treatment group, however, the proportion of women who were satisfied with their treatment did not reach the level of statistical significance. The number of women reporting a change in menstruation was also significantly higher in the implant-treated group (Abou-Setta et al. 2013).

The common adverse effects of progestagens are due to hypo-oestrogenemia and include nausea, weight gain, fluid retention, loss of hair, breast tenderness and breakthrough bleeding. Other adverse effects include acne, edema, reduced bone mineral density and reduced high density lipoproteins.

DANAZOLE

Danazole, a isoxazol derivative of 17a-ethinyltestosterone, is an oral androgenic agent. It directly inhibits steroidogenesis and reduces the GnRH pulses and, thereby suppresses the hypothalamic-pituitary-ovarian axis. It prevents midcycle LH surge and, therefore, ovulation is prevented (Shaw 1992). It also increases metabolic clearance of oestradiol and progesterone, and interacts with endometrial androgen and progesterone receptors. Low estrogen concentration caused by danazole is associated with increased androgen levels (Rotondi et al. 2002; Valle et al. 2003). Hence, it creates an environment that does not support the growth of endometriosis. The amenorrhea resulting from hormonal changes prevents new seeding of implants from the uterus into the peritoneal cavity.

Danazole is administered at a doses ranging from 200-800 mg/day and its efficacy varies with dose. Amenorrhea is considered a good indicator of efficacy. The pain relieving efficacy of danazole is comparable to that of MPA and GnRH analogues. When administered at a dose of 800 mg, its efficacy in decreasing the extent of endometriotic implants is comparable to GnRH analogues (Tummon et al. 1989). The tolerability to danazole, however, is poor compared to GnRH analogues

(Telimaa et al. 1987b; Rotondi et al. 2002). Use of vaginal danazole at a dose of 200 mg/day over 6-12 months in women with recurrent rectovaginal endometriosis was found to be highly effective in relieving endometriosis related pain. Vaginal danazole is also not associated with significant adverse effects (Razzi et al. 2007).

The poor tolerability that results from androgenic and anabolic effects is the major limitation of treatment with oral danazole. The adverse effects of danazole that primarily include weight gain, edema, myalgia, muscle cramps, atrophic breast changes, vasomotor symptoms, acne, oily skin, hirsutism, voice changes and lipid changes limit its use to 6 months. The incidence and severity of adverse effects reduce with reduction of daily doses. One of the open-label randomized controlled trial has shown that 9 month long therapy with 50 mg/day doses of danazole is as effective as GnRH analogues in reducing the endometriosis related pain and menstrual blood loss. Side-effects were observed in 62% of the women but did not lead to treatment withdrawal (Vercellini et al. 1994).

Women on treatment with danazole should use effective contraceptives during the entire period of treatment because of its androgenic effects on the foetus. Use of danazole is contraindicated in women with liver disease because it is largely metabolized in the liver and may cause hepatocellular damage. It is also contraindicated in patients with hypertension, congestive heart failure, or impaired renal function because it can cause fluid retention.

NEWER TREATMENT OPTIONS

Aromatase Inhibitors

Aromatase inhibitors are inhibitors of estrogen biosynthesis. Estrogen biosynthesis requires catalytic conversion of androstenedione and testosterone to estrone and estradiol. The key enzyme required for this reaction is aromatase. Under normal conditions there is no detectable level of aromatase activity in the endometrium.

However, in the endometriotic tissue the activity of this enzyme is induced by inflammatory mediator prostaglandin E_2 to enhance local estrogen production in the diseased implants. Aromatase inhibitors antagonize the actions of aromatase; reduce the local production of estrogen and hence the growth of endometriotic implants (Bulun et al. 2004). Aromatase inhibitors, however, also reduce the estrogen production by ovaries and, therefore, add back therapy using estrogen is required to alleviate the adverse effects due to hypoestrogenemia. Since aromatase inhibitors reduce the estrogen levels, the GnRH secretion increases and causes stimulation of ovarian functions. Therefore, when administered to women of reproductive age group, aromatase inhibitors should be combined with COCPs or progestagens to suppress ovarian functions.

Two prospective studies have demonstrated that the administration of aromatase inhibitors, letrozole or anastrozole, quickly reduces the severity of endometriosis related pain symptoms (Remorgida et al. 2007a; Remorgida et al 2007b). However, recurrence of pain symptoms occurred immediately after the cessation of treatment (Remorgida et al. 2007a). Aromatase inhibitors are also not effective in suppressing the rectovaginal endometriotic lesions. Addition of letrozole to norethindrone acetate, although, produces significant pain relief, it is expensive and causes more adverse effect (Ferrero et al. 2009). Anastrozole (1 mg/day) when given in combination with GnRH analogue over 24 months to women undergone surgical excision, prevention of recurrence has been shown to be better than GnRH analogue given alone (Soysal et al. 2004).

Most of the clinical studies have evaluated the efficacy of aromatase inhibitors in short-term administration (6 months) as the safety of long-term administration in premenopausal women is not established. The common adverse effects caused by aromatase inhibitors include joint pain and myalgia. These agents may also cause headache and gastrointestinal symptoms. The use of aromatase inhibitors in the treatment of endometriosis should be limited to patients who have severe pain persisting despite the use of other medical treatments and surgery.

Selective estrogen receptor modifiers

Selective estrogen receptor modifiers (SERMs) are non-steroidal agents that have affinity for estrogen recptors. However, whether they act as estrogen receptor agonist or antagonist, depends on the target tissue. For the treatment of endometriosis, the SERM that can act as antagonist in endometrium and agonist in bones and lipoproteins may be beneficial. One such agent, TZ-5323, has been shown to have antiestrogenic effects on endometrium. It dose-dependently inhibits the estradiol-stimulated transcriptional activation of estrogen receptors and inhibits binding of estradiol with estrogen receptors. It has shown anti-estrogenic effects in rats without affecting the bone mass. Its beneficial effects for the treatment of human endometriosis have not been investigated.

Selective Progesterone receptor modulators

Selective progesterone receptor modifiers (SPRMs), like SERMs, have affinity for progesterone receptors. However their receptor mediated action, agonism or antagonism, depends on the target tissue. These agents suppress the growth of endometriotic tissue in estrogenic environment, hence their use is not associated with adverse effects due to hypoestrogenemia. Several APRMs have been investigated, however, their benefits need assessment in clinical trials.

Other investigational agents

The following drug classes are still under investigation for therapeutic uses in endometriosis (Ferrero et al. 2010):

1. Immunomodulatory agents: Pentoxifylline, loxorabine, interferon a2b, tumour necrosis factor (TNF)a inhibitors (pentoxifylline, leflunomide, etanercept, infliximab, recombinant human TNF binding protein-I) and interleukin 12.

2. Angiogenesis inhibitors: Inhibitors of vascular endothelial growth factor, TNP470, endostatin, anginex, rapamycin, thalidomide.

3. Matrix metalloproteinase inhibitors: Marimastat (BB2516), primomastat (CGS27023A), tanomastat (ONO4817).

4. Oestrogen receptor β agonist: ERB-041 (selective oestrogen receptor β agonist).

5. Selective oestrogen receptor modulators: Raloxifene.

6. Hypocholesterolemic agents: Probucol, statins (mevastatin, simvastatin, mevalonic acid)

NEWER SYSTEMS FOR HORMONAL DELIVERY

Several new drug delivery systems such as transdermal patch and intravaginal ring may be of benefit in the treatment of endometriosis. They provide sustained drug delivery over longer period of time, however, both of these delivery systems have not been investigated specifically for endometriosis.

A transdermal patch of 20 cm^2 applied on the skin of buttocks, abdomen, upper outer arm or upper torso (excluding the breast) delivers an average daily dose of 150 µg norelgestromin (the active metabolite of norgestimate) and 20 µg ethinyl estradiol into the systemic circulation. It requires weekly replacement. The transdermal patch provides a user-controlled, non-invasive method that allows reduction in the dosing frequency. The patch was shown to provide significantly higher percentage of cycles with perfect dosing compared to that with COCPs (Audet et al. 2001; Archer et al. 2004). However, the efficacy of the patch seems to be affected by body weight (Zieman et al. 2002).

An intravaginal delivery system as a flexible soft, transparent ring also provides a minimally invasive method for hormone delivery. It releases daily doses of 120 µg etonogestrel and 15 µg ethinyl estradiol over a period of 3 weeks and requires monthly replacement. Although, the device has high patient acceptance and better compliance, there is risk of inadvertent expulsion.

CURENT GUIDELINES FOR THE TREATMENT OF

ENDOMETRIOSIS

(Based on European Society of Human reproduction and Embryology, ESHRS, Guidelines 2008)

Several professional organizations have published guidelines for the treatment of endometriosis-related pain and infertility. The recommendations are based on the highest level of available evidences (Table 6). The evidences are graded for their quality using standard criteria as shown in the table 5 below.

Table 5: The Quality of evidence

Level	Evidence
1a	Systematic review and meta-analysis of randomised controlled trials (RCTs)
1b	Evidence obtained from at least one properly randomized controlled trial
2a	Evidence from well-designed controlled trials without randomization
2b	Evidence from at least one other type of well-designed quasi-experimental study
3	Evidence from well-designed, non-experimental, descriptive studies, such as comparative studies, correlation studies or case studies
4	Evidences such as expert committee reports or opinions and/or clinical experience of respected authorities. There is absence of directly applicable clinical studies of good quality.

Table 6. Level of recommendation according to strength of evidence.

Level of recommendation	Strength of evidence
A	Directly based on level 1 evidence
B	Directly based on level 2 evidence or extrapolated recommendation from level 1 evidence
C	Directly based on level 3 evidence or extrapolated recommendation from either level 1 or level 2 evidence
D	Directly based on level 4 evidence or extrapolated recommendation from either level 1, 2 or 3 evidence
GPP	Good practice point based upon the views of the Guideline Development Group

TREATMENT OF PAIN:

1. Empirical treatment of pain symptoms without a definitive diagnosis

GPP	Counselling, adequate analgesia, progestagens, COCPs, and nutritional therapy. The regimen (conventional, continuous or in tricycle) to be followed for the use of COCPs remains unclear. A GnRH agonists may be given but are more expensive, and are associated with more side-effects.

2. Treatment of endometriosis-associated pain in confirmed disease

Non-steroidal anti-inflammatory drugs (NSAIDs)		
A	There is inconclusive evidence to show whether NSAIDs (specifically naproxen) are effective in managing pain caused by endometriosis (Allen et al. 2005).	Evidence level 1a
Hormonal treatment		
A	Suppression of ovarian function for 6 months reduces endometriosis associated pain. The hormonal drugs investigated - COCPs, danazol, gestrinone,	Evidence level 1a

	MPA and GnRH agonists - are equally effective but differ in their side-effect and cost profiles (Davis et al. 2007 ; Prentice et al. 1999; Prentice et al. 2000; Selak et al. 2007). The levonorgestrel intra-uterine system (LNG IUS) also reduces endometriosis associated pain.	
Duration of GnRH treatment		
A	Treatment for 3 months with a GnRH agonist may be as effective as 6 months in terms of pain relief (Hornstein et al. 1995).	Evidence level 1 b
A	When combined with oestrogen and progestagen 'add-back' treatment for up to 2 years appears to be effective and safe in terms of pain relief and bone density protection. Progestagen only 'add-back' is not protective (Sagsveen et al. 2003). However, careful consideration should be given to the use of GnRH agonists in women	Evidence level 1 a

	who may not have reached their maximum bone density.	
Hormone replacement therapy		
C	Hormone replacement therapy (HRT) is recommended after bilateral oophorectomy in young women given the overall health benefits and small risk of recurrent disease while taking HRT (Matorras et al. 2002).	Evidence level 4
	The ideal regimen is unclear: adding a progestagen after hysterectomy is unnecessary but should protect against the unopposed action of oestrogen on any residual disease. However, the theoretical benefit of avoiding disease reactivation and malignant transformation should be balanced against the increase in breast cancer risk reported to be associated with combined oestrogen and progestagen HRT and tibolone (Beral and Million Women Study Collaborators 2003).	
Pre-operative treatment		
A	Although hormonal therapy prior to surgery improves	Evidence level 1a

	Retrospective American Fertility Society Score (rAFS) scores, there is insufficient evidence of any effect on outcome measures such as pain relief (Yap et al. 2004).	
Post-operative treatment		
A	Compared to surgery alone or surgery plus placebo, postoperative hormonal treatment does not produce a significant reduction in pain recurrence at 12 or 24 months, and has no effect on disease recurrence (Yap et al. 2004).	Evidence level 1a

TREATMENT OF ENDOMETRIOSIS-ASSOCIATED INFERTILITY IN CONFIRMED DISEASE

Treatment of endometriotic lesions: Hormonal treatment		
A	Suppression of ovarian function to improve fertility in minimal–mild endometriosis is not effective and should not be offered for this indication alone (Hughes et al. 2007). There is no evidence of its effectiveness in more severe disease.	Evidence level 1a

	Treatment of endometriotic lesions: post-operative treatment	
A	Compared to surgery alone or surgery plus placebo, postoperative hormonal treatment has no effect on pregnancy rates (Yap et al. 2004).	Evidence level 1a
	Assisted reproduction in endometriosis: Intrauterine insemination and in vitro fertilization (IVF)	
A	Treatment with intrauterine insemination (IUI) improves fertility in minimal–mild endometriosis: IUI with ovarian stimulation is effective but the role of unstimulated IUI is uncertain (Tummon et al. 1997).	Evidence level 1b
A	Treatment with a GnRH agonist for 3-6 months before IVF should be considered in women with endometriosis as it increases the odds of clinical pregnancy fourfold. However, the authors of the Cochrane review stressed that the recommendation is based on only one properly randomised study and called for further research, particularly on the mechanism of action (Sallam et al. 2006).	Evidence level 1b
B	Controlled ovarian hyperstimulation (COH) for IVF is equally effective with both GnRH antagonist and	Evidence level 1 b

	GnRH-agonists protocols in terms of implantation and clinical pregnancy rates, but COH with GnRH-a may be preferred because of the availability of more MII oocytes and embryos (Pabuccu et al. 2007).	

References

1. Abou-Setta AM, Houston B, Al-Inany HG, Farquhar C. Levonorgestrel-releasing intrauterine device (LNG-IUD) for symptomatic endometriosis following surgery. Cochrane Database Syst Rev. 2013;1:CD005072.

2. Allen C, Hopewell S, Prentice A, Allen C. Non-steroidal anti-inflammatory drugs for pain in women with endometriosis. Cochrane Database Syst Rev. 2005,4:CD004753.

3. Allen C, Hopewell S, Prentice A, Gregory D. Nonsteroidal anti-inflammatory drugs for pain in women with endometriosis. Cochrane Database Syst Rev. 2009;2:CD004753.

4. American College of Obstetricians and Gynecologists Committee on Practice Bulletins—Gynecology. Medical management of endometriosis. Number 11, December 1999 (replaces Technical Bulletin Number 184, September 1993).

Clinical management guidelines for obstetrician-gynecologists. Int J Gynaecol Obstet 2000;71:183-96.

5. Archer DF, Cullins V, Creasy GW, Fisher AC. The impact of improved compliance with a weekly contraceptive transdermal system (Ortho Evra(R)) on contraceptive efficacy. Contraception. 2004;69:189–95.

6. Audet MC, Moreau M, Koltun WD, Waldbaum AS, Shangold G, Fisher AC, Creasy GW for the ORTHO EVRA/EVRA 004 Study Group. Evaluation of contraceptive efficacy and cycle control of a transdermal contraceptive patch vs an oral contraceptive: a randomized controlled trial. JAMA. 2001;285:2347–54.

7. Barbieri RL. Endometriosis and the estrogen threshold theory. Relation to surgical and medical treatment. J Reprod Med. 1998;43:287-92.

8. Beral V and Million Woman Study Collaborators. Breast cancer and hormone-replacement therapy in the Million Woman Study. Lancet. 2003;362:419-27.

9. Bergqvist A, Theorell T. Changes in quality of life after hormonal treatment of endometriosis. Acta Obstet Gynecol Scand. 2001;80:628-37.

10. Bulun SE, Fang Z, Imir G, Gurates B, Tamura M, Yilmaz B, Langoi D, Amin S, Yang S, Deb S. Aromatase and endometriosis. Semin Reprod Med. 2004;22,45–50.

11. Bulun SE. Endometriosis. N Engl J Med. 2009;360:268-79.

12. Cheewadhanaraks S, Choksuchat C, Dhanaworavibul K, Liabsuetrakul T. Postoperative depot medroxyprogesterone acetate versus continuous oral contraceptive pills in the treatment of endometriosis-associated pain: a randomized comparative trial. Gynecol Obstet Invest. 2012;74(2):151-6.

13. Child TJ, Tan SL. Endometriosis: aetiology, pathogenesis and treatment. Drugs. 2001;61:1735–50.

14. Chwalisz K, Surrey E, Stanczyk FZ. The hormonal profile of norethindrone acetate: rationale for add-back therapy with gonadotropin-releasing hormone agonists in women with endometriosis. Reprod Sci. 2012;19(6):563-71.

15. Cirkel U, Ochs H, Schneider HPG. A randomized, comparative trial of triptorelin depot (D-Trp6-LHRH) and danazol in the treatment of endometriosis. Eur J Obstet Gynecol Reprod Biol. 1995;59:61–9.

16. Cosson M, Querleu D, Donnez J, et al. Dienogest is as effective as triptorelin in the treatment of endometriosis after laparoscopic surgery: Results of a prospective, multicenter, randomized study. Fertil Steril. 2002;77(4):684–92.

17. Crosignani PG, Luciano A, Ray A, Bergqvist A. Subcutaneous depot medroxyprogesterone acetate versus leuprolide acetate in the treatment of endometriosis-associated pain. Hum Reprod 2006a;21:248-56.

18. Crosignani PG, Olive D, Bergqvist A, Luciano A. Advances in the management of endometriosis: an update for clinicians. Human Reproduction Update. 2006b;12(2):179–89.

19. Davis L, Kennedy SS, Moore J, Prentice A. Modern combined oral contraceptives for pain associated with endometriosis (Cochrane Review). Cochrane Database Syst Rev. 2007;3:CD001019.

20. Fedele L, Bianchi S, Marchini M, Di Nola G. Histological impact of medical therapy--clinical implications. Br J Obstet Gynaecol. 1995;102(Suppl 12):8-11.

21. Ferrero S, Abbamonte LH, Parisi M, et al. Dyspareunia and quality of sex life after laparoscopic excision of endometriosis and postoperative administration of triptorelin. Fertil Steril. 2007;87:227-9.

22. Ferrero S, Camerini G, Seracchioli R, et al. Letrozole combined with norethisterone acetate compared with norethisterone acetate alone in the treatment of pain symptoms caused by endometriosis. Hum Reprod. 2009;24:3033-41.

23. Ferrero S, Remorgida V, Venturini PL. Current pharmacotherapy for endometriosis. Expert Opin Pharmacother. 2010;11(7):1123-34.

24. Franke HR, van de Weijer PH, Pennings TM, van der Mooren MJ. Gonadotropin-releasing hormone agonist plus "add-back" hormone replacement therapy for treatment of endometriosis: a prospective, randomized, placebo-controlled, double-blind trial. Fertil Steril. 2000;74:534-9.

25. Fraser IS, Shearman RP, Jansen RPS, Sutherland PD. A comparative treatment trial of endometriosis using the gonadotrophin-releasing hormone agonist, nafarelin, and the synthetic steroid, danazol. Aust N Z J Obstet Gynaecol. 1991;31:158–63.

26. Gestrinone Italian Study Group. Gestrinone versus a gonadotropin-releasing hormone agonist for the treatment of pelvic pain associated with endometriosis: a multicenter, randomized, double-blind study. Fertil Steril. 1996;66:911-9.

27. Halis G, Mechsner S, Ebert AD. The Diagnosis and Treatment of Deep infiltrating Endometriosis. Dtsch Arztebl Int. 2010;107(25):446–56.

28. Harada T, Momoeda M, Taketani Y, Hoshiai H, Terakawa N. Low-dose oral contraceptive pill for dysmenorrhea associated

with endometriosis: a placebo-controlled, double-blind, randomized trial. Fertil Steril. 2008;90(5):1583–8.

29. Harada T, Momoeda M, Taketani Y, et al. Dienogest is as effective as intranasal buserelin acetate for the relief of pain symptoms associated with endometriosis – a randomized, double-blind, multicenter, controlled trial. Fertil Steril. 2009;91(3):675–81.

30. Harrison RF, Barry-Kinsella C. Efficacy of medroxyprogesterone treatment in infertile women with endometriosis: a prospective, randomized, placebo-controlled study. Fertil Steril. 2000;74:24-30.

31. Hee L, Kettner LO, Vejtorp M. Continuous use of oral contraceptives: an overview of effects and side-effects. Acta Obstet Gynecol Scand. 2013;92(2):125-36.

32. Hornstein MD, Yuzpe AA, Burry KA, Heinrichs LR, Buttram-VL J, Orwoll ES. Prospective randomized double-blind trial of 3 versus 6 months of nafarelin therapy for endometriosis associated pelvic pain. Fertil Steril. 1995;63:955-62.

33. Hornstein MD, Hemmings R, Yuzpe AA, Heinrichs WL. Use of nafarelin versus placebo after reductive laparoscopic surgery for endometriosis. Fertil Steril. 1997;68:860-4.

34. Hughes E, Fedorkow D, Collins J, Vandekerckhove P. Ovulation suppression for endometriosis. Cochrane Database Syst Rev. 2007;3:CD000155.

35. Köhler G, Faustmann TA, Gerlinger C, Seitz C, Mueck AO. A dose-ranging study to determine the efficacy and safety of 1, 2, and 4mg of dienogest daily for endometriosis. Int J Gynaecol Obstet. 2010;108(1):21-5.

36. Loverro G, Carriero C, Rossi AC, et al. A randomized study comparing triptorelin or expectant management following conservative laparoscopic surgery for symptomatic stage III-IV endometriosis. Eur J Obstet Gynecol Reprod Biol. 2008;136:194-8.

37. Matorras R, Elorriage MA, Pijoan JI, Ramon O, Rodriguez-Escudero FJ. Recurrence of endometriosis in women with bilateral adnexectomy (with or without total hysterectomy) who received hormone replacement therapy. Fertil Steril. 2002;77:303-8.

38. Moghissi KS, Boyce CR. Management of endometriosis with oral edroxyprogesterone acetate. Obstet Gynecol. 1976;47:265-7.

39. Momoeda M, Taketani Y. Randomized double-blind, multicentre, parallel-group dose–response study of dienogest in

patients with endometriosis. Jpn Pharmacol Ther. 2007;35:769–83.

40. Momoeda M, Harada T, Terakawa N, et al. Long-term use of dienogest for the treatment of endometriosis. J Obstet Gynaecol Res. 2009;35(6):1069–76.

41. Muneyyirci-Delale O, Anopa J, Charles C, Mathur D, Parris R, Cutler JB, Salame G, Abulafia O. Medical management of recurrent endometrioma with long-term norethindrone acetate. Int J Women's Health. 2012;4:149–54.

42. Pabuccu R, Onalan G, Kaya C. GnRH agonist and antagonist protocols for stage I-II endometriosis and endometrioma in in vitro fertilization/intracytoplasmic sperm injection cycles. Fertil. Steril. 007;88(4),832–9.

43. Petraglia F, Hornung D, Seitz C, et al. Reduced pelvic pain in women with endometriosis: efficacy of long-term dienogest treatment. Arch Gynecol Obstet. 2012;285(1):167–73.

44. Petta CA, Ferriani RA, Abrao MS, et al. Randomized clinical trial of a levonorgestrel-releasing intrauterine system and a depot GnRH analogue for the treatment of chronic pelvic pain in women with endometriosis. Hum Reprod. 2005;20:1993-8.

45. Prentice A, Deary AJ, Goldbeck WS, Farquhar C, Smith SK. Gonadotrophin-releasing hormone analogues for pain associated

with endometriosis (Cochrane Review). The Cochrane Database Syst Rev. 1999;2CD000346.

46. Prentice A, Deary AJ, Bland E. Progestagens and anti-progestagens for pain associated with endometriosis. Cochrane Database Syst Rev. 2000;2:CD002122.

47. Razzi S, Luisi S, Calonaci F, Altomare A, Bocchi C, Petraglia F. Efficacy of vaginal danazol treatment in women with recurrent deeply infiltrating endometriosis. Fert Steril. 2007;88(4):789-94.

48. Remorgida V, Abbamonte HL, Ragni N, et al. Letrozole and norethisterone acetate in rectovaginal endometriosis. Fertil Steril. 2007a;88:724-6.

49. Remorgida V, Abbamonte LH, Ragni N, et al. Letrozole and desogestrel-only contraceptive pill for the treatment of stage IV endometriosis. Aust NZ J Obstet Gynaecol. 2007b;47:222-5.

50. Roland M, Leisten D, Kane RJ. Endometriosis therapy with medroxyprogesterone acetate. Reprod Med. 1976;17:249-52.

51. Rotondi M, Labriola D, Rotondi M, Ammaturo FP, Amato G, Carella C, Izzo A, Panariello S. Depot leuprorelin acetate versus danazol in the treatment of infertile women with symptomatic endometriosis. Eur J Gynaecol Oncol. 2002;23:523–6.

52. Sagsveen M, Farmer JE, Prentice A, Breeze A. Gonadotrophin-releasing hormone analogues for endometriosis: bone mineral

density (Cochrane Review). Cochrane Database Syst Rev. 2003;4: CD001297.

53. Sallam HN, Garcia-Velasco JA, Dias S, Arici A. Long-term pituitary down-regulation before in vitro fertilization (IVF) for women with endometriosis. Cochrane Database Syst Rev. 2006;1:CD004635.

54. Schindler AE, Campagnoli C, Druckmannc R, Huber J, Pasqualini JR, Schweppef KW, Thijssen JHH. Classification and pharmacology of progestins. Maturitas. 2003;46S1:S7–S16.

55. Selak V, Farquhar C, Prentice A, Singla A. Danazol for pelvic pain associated with endometriosis. Cochrane Database Systc Rev. 2007;4:CD000068.

56. Seracchioli R, Mabrouk M, Frasca` C, et al. Long-term oral contraceptive pills and postoperative pain management after laparoscopic excision of ovarian endometrioma: a randomized controlled trial. Fertil Steril. 2010;94(2):464-71.

57. Shaw RW. Treatment of endometriosis. Lancet 1992;340:1267-71.

58. Soysal S, Soysal ME, Ozer S, et al. The effects of post-surgical administration of goserelin plus anastrozole compared to goserelin alone in patients with severe endometriosis: a prospective randomized trial. Hum Reprod. 2004;19:160-7.

59. Strowitzki T, Faustmann T, Gerlinger C, Seitz C. Dienogest in the treatment of endometriosis-associated pelvic pain: A 12-week, randomized, double-blind, placebo-controlled study. Eur J Obstet Gynecol Reprod Biol. 2010a;151(2):193–8.

60. Strowitzki T, Marr J, Gerlinger C, Faustmann T, Seitz C. Dienogest is as effective as leuprolide acetate in treating the painful symptoms of endometriosis: A 24-week, randomized, multicentre, open-label trial. Hum Reprod. 2010b;25(3):633–41.

61. Telimaa S, Puolakka J, Rönnberg L, Kauppila A. Placebo-controlled comparison of danazol and high-dose medroxyprogesterone acetate in the treatment of endometriosis. Gynecol Endocrinol 1987a;1:13-23.

62. Telimaa S, Rönnberg L, Kauppila A. Placebo-controlled comparison of danazol and high-dose medroxyprogesterone acetate in the treatment of endometriosis after conservative surgery. Gynecol Endocrinol. 1987b;1:363–71.

63. Tummon IS, Asher LJ, Martin JS, Tulandi T. Randomized controlled trial of superovulation and insemination for infertility associated with minimal or mild endometriosis. Fertil Steril. 1997;68:8-12.

64. Tummon IS, Pepping ME, Binor Z, et al. A randomized, prospective comparison of endocrine changes induced with

intranasal leuprolide or danazol for treatment of endometriosis. Fertil Steril 1989;51:390-4.

65. Valle RF, Sciarra JJ. Endometriosis: treatment strategies. Ann N Y Acad Sci. 2003;997:229–39.

66. Van Gorp T, Amant F, Neven P, Vergote I, Moeman P. Endometriosis and the development of malignant tumours of the pelvis. A review of literature. Best Pract Res Clin Obstet Gynaecol 2004;18(2):349-71.

67. Vercellini P, Trespidi L, Colombo A, et al. A gonadotropin-releasing hormone agonist versus a low-dose oral contraceptive for pelvic pain associated with endometriosis. Fertil Steril. 1993;60:75-9.

68. Vercellini P, Trespidi L, Panazza S, et al. Very low dose danazol for relief of endometriosis-associated pelvic pain: a pilot study. Fertil Steril. 1994;62:1136-42.

69. Vercellini P, De Giorgi O, Oldani S, et al. Depot medroxyprogesterone acetate versus an oral contraceptive combined with very-low-dose danazol for long-term treatment of pelvic pain associated with endometriosis. Am J Obstet Gynecol. 1996;175:396-401.

70. Vercellini P, De Giorgi O, Mosconi P, et al. Cyproterone acetate versus a continuous monophasic oral contraceptive in the

treatment of recurrent pelvic pain after conservative surgery for symptomatic endometriosis. Fertil Steril. 2002;77:52-61.

71. Vercellini P, Frontino G, De Giorgi O, Aimi G, Zaina B, Crosignani PG. Comparison of a levonorgestrel-releasing intrauterine device versus expectant management after conservative surgery for symptomatic endometriosis: a pilot study. Fertil Steril. 2003;80(2):305-9.

72. Vercellini P, Pietropaolo G, De Giorgi O, et al. Treatment of symptomatic rectovaginal endometriosis with an estrogen-progestogen combination versus low-dose norethindrone acetate. Fertil Steril. 2005;84:1375-87.

73. Winkel CA. Evaluation and management of women with endometriosis. Obstet Gynecol. 2003;102(2):397-408.

74. Yap C, Furness S, Farquhar C. Pre and post operative medical therapy for endometriosis surgery. Cochrane Database Syst Rev. 2004;3CD003678.

75. Zieman M, Guillebaud J, Weisberg E, Shangold GA, Fisher AC, Creasy GW. Contraceptive efficacy and cycle control with the Ortho Evra™/Evra™ transdermal system: the analysis of pooled data. Fertil Steril. 2002;77:S13–S18.

10 ENDOMETRIOSIS AND FUTURE DIRECTIONS

Although, since the original clinical depiction of endometriosis, much has been achieved in enhancing our understanding of this debilitating disease. Whereas no one theory of pathogenesis can account for all of the defined manifestations of endometriosis, the retrograde menstruation theory is widely acknowledged to account for the dissemination of endometrial cells. What awaits to be explored is the identification of the specific factor or factors that synchronise the survival and consequent implantation of the displaced endometrium. A proposal had beem put up to look into this area of research in order to help both in the noninvasive diagnosis as well as shed light on some aspect of the pathogenesis of endometriosis.

Areas of interest are centered around elucidation of the formation of endometriotic implants and this would embrace exploration of intrinsic or acquired attributes of the endometrium and faulty immune clearance apropos endometriotic implants. Variation especially in lesional phenotype, warrants histopathologic validation of implants in clinical and molecular research. Research should also focus on the disease heterogeneity. The foundations emblematic of inflammation, estrogen dependence, and progesterone resistance in the pathophysiology of endometriosis-related pain and infertility are fertile fields for dynamic research. Greater advances in our understanding of endometriosis, preventive strategies, novel non-surgical diagnostic modalities and targeted therapeutics offer great promise for optimistic future. A comprehensive comprehension of the histopathogenesis and pathophysiology of endometriosis is vital for the development of novel diagnostic and treatment approaches for this debilitating condition [1].

There is great scope for large well controlled clinical studies comprising women with and without endometriosis as the cause of infertility and pain and women with and without inferrility and pain [2]. It is essential to have control groups in clinical studies and multicenter randomised trials.

Pharmacological

- management of

- endometriosis must be set within the framework of long-term therapeutic strategies.

- Combined oral contraceptives and progestins are recommended as the first-line option, both as an alternative to surgery and as a postoperative adjuvant measure..There is no indication for medical treatment in women seeking conception because reproductive

- prognosis is not ameliorated [3].

11. Administration of TNF binding protei

14. ns to block TNF alpha activity, at the same time as one injects menstrual endometrium, then one can hamper to a great extent the the development of endometriosis in baboons. Moreover, one can fully prevent the development of endometriosis-related adhesions [2]. With new advances

16. in the understanding of pathophysiology of endometriosis, it is being considered as an autoimmune disorder. Novel therapies using immunomodulators and other novel compounds are recommended.. An ideal drug would be one that treats endometriosis without hampering fertility [4].

It is appraised that the exorbitant annual cost of endometriosis exceeds US $12 000 per woman.This cost includes one-third of the direct health care costs with two-thirds ascribed to loss of productivity.

While admittedly decreased quality of life is the most significant forecaster of direct health care total costs matter very much. Apart from this the issue is compounded by the unfortunate delay ,(a mean delay of 6.7 years) between start of symptoms and a surgical diagnosis of endometriosis, each afflicted subject loses on average 10.8 hours of work weekly, mostly due to reduced work efficiency. In order to foster and facilitate research into this devastating disease, a consensus workshop to define future directions for endometriosis research was conducted in conjunction with the 11th World Congress on Endometriosis in September 2011 in Montpellier, France. This workshop aimed to review and update the endometriosis research priorities consensus statement developed after the 10th World Congress on Endometriosis in 2008 [5]. There were 56 recommendations for research that have been developed, and grouped under 6 subheadings: (1) diagnosis, (2) classification andprognosis, (3) clinical trials, treatment, and outcomes, (4) epidemiology, (5) pathophysiology, and (6) research policy. It is hoped that this consensus international research priorities blue print of the workshop participants and researchers will be empowered and encouraged to develop new interdisciplinary research proposals that will enhance funding support for work on endometriosis [5].

Future research in endometriosis should focus on pathogenesis studies in the baboon model, the early interactions between endometrial and peritoneal cells in the pelvic cavity at the time of menstruation, and posible differences between eutopic endometrium and myometrium in women with and without endometriosis [2]. The baboon model of endometriosis is enormously valauable to explore the pathogenesis and evolution of endometriosis from its beginning to the advanced established disease [6].

The need for more integration between the areas of epidemiology and genetics.is emphasised. Pelvic inflammation in women with endometriosis could be the target for new diagnostic and therapeutic approaches. Many important questions await results apropos the link between endometriosis and environmental factors. Careful analysis of systemic and extrapelvic manifestations of endometriosis, and better tools are required to evalaute quality of life in women with chronic pain caused by endometriosis. Most current evidence supports a causal relationship between endometriosis and subfertility, and the spontaneous progressive nature of endometriosis has been demonstrated in 30% to 60% of patients. Recurrence of endometriosis after classic medical and surgical therapy is a major and underestimated problem, especially in women with advanced disease. It is essential to integrate clinical and research teams that combine expert medical, surgical, and holistic care with state-of-the-art research expertise in immunology, endocrinology, and genetics to discover new diagnostic methods and medical treatments for endometriosis [2].

The failure of inflammatory reaction in the peritoneal cavity at the endometriotic site to eliminate the refluxed endometrial fragments also seems to support the persistence of the tissue favouring the development of the disease. Determination of the interactions between peritoneal macrophages and cytotoxic T cells and endometrial cells may help shed more light on their scavenging ability and impact on the state of apoptosis. It is paramount to delineate the mechanism(s) underlying induction of the expression of estrogen and its receptor (ERβ) for clearer comprehension of the evolvement of endometriosis. Study of the impact of ERβ activation in endometriotic lesions is warranted.as much as it is important to investigate the effects of estrogen on the role of the immune cells, either directly or indirectly. Exploring the effect of events at sites of ectopic endometrium on the eutopic endometrium may explain the mechanism(s) of infertility linked with endometriosis [6].

Nnoaham and collaborators 2011 [7], estimated the effect of endometriosis on health-related quality of life (HRQoL) and work productivity conducted a multicenter cross-sectional study with prospective recruitment. The study comprised sixteen clinical centers in ten countries with a total of 1,418 premenopausal women, aged 18-45 years, without a previous surgical diagnosis of endometriosis, having laparoscopy to investigate symptoms or to be sterilized. The study concluded that endometriosis diminishes HRQoL and work productivity transcending borders across countries and ethnicities. it was amply clear that a high index of suspicion is essential to hasten specialist assessment of symptomatic women. Future research should focus on elucidating pain mechanisms relating to severity of endometriosis [7].

A study was performed to verify the hypothesis that vitamins C, E, and the B vitamins may affect factors implicated in the pathogenesis of endometriosis, such as oxidative stress andsteroid hormone metabolism [8]. Researchers examined the relation between intake of vitamins C, E, the B vitamins, and the use of multivitamin supplements and diagnosis of endometriosis. The study entailed collection of data from 1383 incident cases of laparoscopically-confirmed endometriosis in the Nurses' Health Study II between1991 and 2005. Diet was assessed via food frequency questionnaire. Incidence rate ratios (RR) and 95% confidence intervals (CI) were estimated using time-varying Cox proportional hazards models.The study concluded that thiamine, folate, vitamin C, and vitamin E from food sources are inversely linked to endometriosis risk. The protective mechanism may not be associated with the nutrients perse instead other constituents of foods abundant in these micronutrients or factors correlated with diets high in these vitamin-rich foods [8].

It is open to further research to investigate into this aspect to unravel the factors correlating with diets abundant in thses virtamin rich foods. The health benefits of Green tea, the most popular beverage, has been recognised for a long time, and now it is credited with its potency to control endometriosis [9]. Researchers at the Chinese University of Hong

Kong have established that catechins, or potent antioxidant compounds in green tea, restricts angiogenesis, which contributes to the spread of endometriosis [9].

An investigation to verify the validity of the premise that consumption of dairy foods, nutrients in women with endometriosis was conducted [10]. The study comprised 1385 cases of incident laparoscopically confirmed endometriosis in Nurses' Health Study II. Diet was assessed via food frequency questionnaire. Intakes of total and low-fat dairy foods were associated with a lower risk of endometriosis. The findings suggest that higher predicted plasma 25(OH)D levels and higher intake of dairy foods are related to a decreased risk of endometriosi [10].

There is a pressing need to extend the genetic studies now that the techniques are emerging and to make clinical studies available. Agneta Bergqvist) Agneta Bergqvist, explained the background for the 1st JOINT ASRM/ESHRE/APEA MEETING 16 September 2005 in Maastricht which aimed to encourage global collaboration in the field of endometriosis. In this context it is worth mentioning the progress that has been made in this field of research. Prior studies using genomics techniques have established gene products are abnormally expressed in endometriotic tissues. Additionally, novel transcripts previously unappreciated in endometriosis were discovered. Dysregulated genes in endometriosis include glycodelin, complement, early growth response-1 and transducer of erbB-1. Global gene profiling studies have immense potential to transform thediagnosis and management of endometriosis and other human diseases [11].

Collaborative studies in academic and pharmaceutical industry genomics techniques have demonstrated abnormal expression of gene products in endometriotic tissues. In addition, novel transcripts which have not been previously appreciated in this condition have been discovered. The spectrum of dysregulated genes in endometriosis includes glycodelin, complement, early growth response-1 and transducer of erbB-1.Global gene profiling studies may shed more light to project a paradigm shift in he diagnosis and treatment of endometriosis and other human diseases [11].

Over the last two decades, several proteomics technologies have been employed to explore serum markers for endometriosis. While some molecules identified by proteomics technologies may be pertinent in the pathogenesis of endometriosis, potential serum markers for this condition are yet to be discovered for any clinical application [12].

Endometriosis has multifaceted characteristics; most case–control studies have not adhered to the fundamental standard rule of epidemiological study plan. Suitable choice of control is problematic. A properly planned case control study will serve as an appropriate substitute to the prospective cohort study. It is more desirable to utilise newly diagnosed cases than prevalent ones because the latter may change risk assessments and confound the analysis of findings. Controls must be carefully chosen from the source population composing the cases. It is imperative to look into possible confusion both in studies of environmental and genetic factors. As regards endometriosis, a suggested study strategy would be to: (i) include recently diagnosed cases with `endometriosis (ii) gather facts preceding onset of symptom and (iii) include at least one population-based female control group matched on unadjustable confounders and screened for pelvic symptoms. Future studies of endometriosis have to integrate both environmental and genetic factors Appropriately planned studies will ensure reliable results and aid identification of any real aetiologic heterogeneity anticipated in a complex trait [13].

It is known that endometriosis is linked with loss of heterozygosity (LOH) at the *10q23.3* locus, *PTEN* somatic mutations and alterations in the levels and sharing of proteins in the PTEN-PI3K/Akt signal transduction pathway. The study was performed to verify if mutations in the phosphatase and tensin homolog deleted on chromosome 10 (*PTEN*) gene are related to endometriosis. Current genome-wide association and linkage studies have reported noteworthy connection of endometriosis with *7p15.2, 9p21* and *10q23-26* loci. *PTEN*, which maps to *10q23.3*, acts as a tumor suppressor gene via the action of its phosphatase protein product, phosphatase and tensin homolog (PTEN) [14]. This case control study enrolled a total of 1252 subjects of Indian origin (endometriosis patients = 752; controls = 500) from 2001 to 2009, India [14]. PCR-GeneScan analysis revealed a greater LOH frequency at *10q23.3* (84.4%) compared with other loci hence they concentrated on *PTEN*. PCR-sequencing analysis which exhibited seven novel somatic mutations and 23 germ-line polymorphisms in patients. Amongst somatic mutations, a frame-shift insertion at 10:89692992–89692993 (in the functionally important N-terminal phosphatase domain of PTEN) happened in 11 of the 32 ectopic endometria. Western-blot and immunohistochemical analysis showed reduced PTEN and elevated p-Akt and p-Bad levels in eutopic endometria of patients in comarison with controls. Additionally , PTEN loss was more common in the nucleus than in the cytoplasm. There was no difference in expression of p27 between patients and controls. Their results signified a potential participation of the PTEN-PI3K/Akt-Bad axis in the pathogenesis of endometriosis, which may unravel appropriate pathway inhibitors for treatemnt of endometriosi [14]. The investigators recommended that future studies should included a bigger sample size and analysis of the role of the other genes involved in the PTEN-PI3K/Akt signal transduction pathway [14].

References

1. Richard O. Burney, M.Sc. and Linda C. Giudice. Pathogenesis and Pathophysiology of Endometriosis. Fertil Steril. 2012; 98(3): 10.

2. D'Hooghe TM, Debrock S, Meuleman C, Hill JA, Mwenda JM. Future directions in endometriosis research. Obstet Gynecol Clin North Am. 2003;30(1):221-44

3. Paolo Vercellini,

Endometriosis: current and future medical therapies. Best Practice &

Research Clinical Obstetrics & Gynaecology 2008; 22(2): 275–306.

4. Harmeet Malhotra. New Developments in Medical Management of Endometriosis. Apollo Medicine 2009; 3: 247–25.

5. Rogers PA, D'Hooghe TM, Fazleabas A, Giudice LC, Montgomery GW, Petraglia F,Taylor RN. Defining future directions for endometriosis research: workshop report from the 2011 World Congress of Endometriosis In Montpellier, France. Reprod Sci. 2013;20(5): 483-99.

6. Julie M. Hastings, Asgerally T. Fazleabas Future Directions in Endometriosis. Research Semin Reprod Med 2003; 21(2): 255-262

7. Nnoaham KE, Hummelshoj L, Webster P, d'Hooghe T, de Cicco Nardone F, de Cicco Nardone C, Jenkinson C, Kennedy SH, Zondervan KT; World Endometriosis Research Foundation Global Study of Women's Health consortium. Impact of endometriosis on quality of life and work productivity: a multicenterstudy across ten countries. Fertil Steril. 2011;96(2): 366-373.

8. Darling AM, Chavarro JE, Malspeis S, Harris HR, Missmer SA. A prospective cohort study of Vitamins B, C, E, and multivitamin intake andendometriosis. A prospective cohort study of Vitamins B, C, E, and multivitamin intake andendometriosis. J Endometr. 2013; 5(1):17-26.

9. Xu H, Becker CM, Lui WT, Chu CY, Davis TN, Kung AL, Birsner AE, D'Amato RJ, Wai Man GC, Wang CC. Green tea epigallocatechin-3-gallate inhibits angiogenesis and suppresses vascular endothelial growth factor C/vascular endothelial growth factor receptor 2 expression and signaling in experimental endometriosis in vivo. Fertil Steril. 2011; 96(4):1021-8.

10. Harris HR, Chavarro JE, Malspeis S, Willett WC, Missmer SA. Dairy-food, calcium, magnesium, and vitamin D intake and endometriosis: a prospective cohort study. Am J Epidemiol. 2013 ;177(5): 420-30.

11. Taylor RN, Lundeen SG, Giudice LC. Emerging role of genomics in endometriosis research. Fertil Steril. 2002;78(4): 694-8.

12. Ferrero S, Gillott DJ, Remorgida V, Ragni N, Venturini PL, Grudzinskas JG. Proteomics technologies in endometriosis. Expert Rev Proteomics. 2008; 5(5):705-14.

13. Krina T. Zondervan, Lon R. Cardon and Stephen H. Kennedy. Design issues for complex traits such as endometriosis What makes a good case–control study? Hum. Reprod. 2002; 17 (6): 1415-1423.

14. Suresh Govatati, Vijaya Lakshmi Kodati, Mamata Deenadayal, Baidyanath Chakravarty, Sisinthy Shivaji and Manjula Bhanoori, Mutations in the *PTEN* tumor gene and risk of endometriosis: a case–control study Hum. Reprod. 2014; 29 (2): 324-336.

ABOUT THE AUTHORS

Dr. Methil Kannan Kutty; FRCP, presently is Professor of Pathology in Faculty of Medicine, Univesiti Teknologi MARA Malaysia. He has held Professor of Pathology in University Islam Malaysia, UKM Malaysia, International Medical University Malaysia, Royal college of Medicine, and King Faisal University, Dammam, KSA. He is the author of five books and he has published more than 150 papers in peer reviewed journals.

Dr. Muhamed T. Osman; PhD, presently, is Associate Professor of Pathology in Faculty of Medicine and Defence Health, National Defence University of Malaysia. He was Consultant Pathologist and Clinical Lecturer at Teaching Laboratories at Medical City of Baghdad, Iraq and Senior Lecturer of Pathology at UiTM Malaysia. He is the author of five books and has published more than 60 papers in peer reviewed journals.

www.ingramcontent.com/pod-product-compliance
Lightning Source LLC
Chambersburg PA
CBHW051440170526
45166CB00001B/55